Safer Hanc
People in the
Community

Produced by

BackCare
The National Organisation for Healthy Backs

the new name for the National Back Pain Association

We wish to thank The Colt Foundation for their generous support in the production of this handbook.

Published by BackCare the new name for National Back Pain Association, 16 Elmtree Road, Teddington, Middlesex TW11 8ST. Registered Charity No. 256751

Foreword

When people injured their backs in the 1960s there was less known and understood about back pain than there is today; back injury ended the careers of thousands of people every year. The pain and disability suffered was immense. Since then the work of the National Back Pain Association, now BackCare, has been dedicated to addressing the appalling incidence of back injuries and illnesses in Britain. We became aware of the dangers of back injury through lifting that nurses faced every day in the course of their work, and this led us to call together a team of experts to develop and publish the first edition of the Guide to the Handling of Patients in 1981. Little did we know that our book would become the standard training text in the National Health Service, updated a further three times, with the publication of the fourth edition in 1997.

Handling training and hospital equipment has become more sophisticated, and the recent fourth edition of the Guide reflects this change. While earlier editions were used in many residential and care homes, Care Managers and Care Staff in the community began to tell us about their need for a manual geared more closely to the very different settings in which they work. In response to this, BackCare brought together an expert writing team dedicated to helping us produce SAFER HANDLING OF PEOPLE IN THE COMMUNITY. We hope both Care Managers and Care Staff will find in this book a valuable source of information and advice.

We urge you to remember that the book is written for your benefit. When you go to work each day you take your back with you. Used well, the guidance in these pages can help you to look after your own back and save a great deal of suffering. But safer handling does not stop in the training room; it does not stop with this book! It is something that needs to be thought about all the time.

If we can offer you a simple motto to keep in mind every day it is 'Think BACK before you ACT'.

With best wishes

Sir Frank Davies, CBE OStJ
Chairman of the Health and Safety Commission
Chairman of BackCare

Contents

Contributors

Co-ordinating Author

Ron Steed BScN, RGN Cert. Ed. Consultant Back Care Adviser and Back Care Adviser for Back to Safety Ltd., Walmer, Deal, Kent

Editor

Liz Aitchison, MA, CQSW, Chief Officer, Age Concern Kingston upon Thames

Authors

Sally Cassar, MCSP, Dip. H.Ed, Dip. T.P., Freelance Consultant Manual Handling Adviser and Trainer

Joyce Cheney, MCSP, Cert. Ed. Manual Handling Co-ordinator, Kent and Canterbury Hospitals, Canterbury

Julian Pearce, MCSP, MSc, Lecturer in Physiotherapy, School of Occupational Therapy and Physiotherapy, University of Southampton

Kevin Tesh, PhD, MErgs, MIOSH, Senior Ergonomist, Institute of Occupational Medicine, Edinburgh and Ergonomics Adviser to Education Committee of BackCare

Clive Tracey, RGN, DMS, IOSH, Manual Handling Co-ordinator, Kings College Hospital, London and Consultant Back Care Adviser

Sue Wiltshire, RGN, RCNT, Trainer and Risk Assessor, Domiciliary Care, Social Services Dept., London Borough of Richmond upon Thames

Patricia P. Wright, RGN, DN, FECert., Retired Community Nurse Manager and Community Tutor, former Trustee of the NBPA

With thanks to Doreen Field DDCM, DMS, Principal Manager, Domiciliary Care, Social Services Dept., London Borough of Richmond upon Thames for her contribution to Sue Wiltshire's section of Chapter 1.

Index

Jill Dormon BSc (Hons), Accredited Indexer

Design & cover illustration

Karen Penny, Publications Officer, BackCare

Illustrator

Candida Kennedy, Freelance Illustrator

Origination Photography

Gordon Penny, Freelance Photographer

Publisher

BackCare, 16 Elmtree Road, Teddington, Middlesex TW11 8ST

Printed by

Hammond Vivian, Richmond

Acknowledgements

Back Care wishes to acknowledge the invaluable contribution that has been made by a number of people to the preparation of this book. Many individuals have given their time to review chapters, make suggestions and give advice to the authors and the editorial team. We are indebted to them.

Lois Arnold, CQSW, Dip SW, Assistant Team Manager, Cambridgeshire Social Services

Sally Cassar, MCSP, Dip. H. Ed. Dip.T.P., Freelance Consultant Manual Handling Adviser and Trainer

Malcolm Darvill, Head of Ergonomic and Psychosocial Policy Unit, Health and Safety Executive (HSE)

Elaine Fazel, RGN, RM, DMS, FETC, Moving and Handling Co-ordinator, Wigan & Leigh NHS Trust

Jacqui Hall, MSc, RGN, RNT, Cert Ed, NNEB, Cert in Patient Handling and Moving, Senior Lecturer, University of Northumbria at Newcastle

Pat Harding, SROT, T DipCot, Cert Ed FE, Occupational Therapist, British Red Cross, Medical Aid Dept, Leicestershire Disabled Living Centre

Linda de Henau, RGN, BSc (Hons), Cert Ed, Moving and Handling Adviser, East Kent Hospitals NHS Trust

Sheila S Kitchen, PhD, MSc, MCSP, Dip.T.P., Deputy Head, Division of Physiotherapy, Kings College, London

John McElwaine, Manual Handling Policy Co-ordinator, Health Directorate, Health and Safety Executive (HSE)

Rosemary Mills, RN, DMS, MiMgt, Proprietor, The Mills Group of Nursing Homes, Kent

David G J Mullooly, Policy Officer, Health Directorate, Health and Safety Executive (HSE)

Peter Phillips, Media Producer, Teaching Support & Media Services, University of Southampton

Hugh Robertson, Head of Health and Safety, UNISON

Gerard Smale, MA, CQSW, Director of Development, National Institute of Social Work and Visiting Professor, Goldsmith's College, University of London

Nicki Stott, RGN, DN, Cert ONC, Manager/Nurse Adviser, British Red Cross, Medical Aid Dept, Leicestershire Disabled Living Centre

Kevin Tesh, PhD, MErgs, MIOSH, Senior Ergonomist, Institute of Occupational Medicine, Edinburgh and Ergonomics Adviser to Education Committee of BackCare

With special thanks to Ian Jackson for sharing his personal experience with us.

Introduction

Ian Jackson is a 65 year old man with advanced multiple sclerosis (MS) now affecting all his limbs; he has also had his right leg amputated just above the knee in a recent operation. Diagnosed with MS over 22 years ago, Ian has been receiving care for the last 10 years.

"At 6'6" and around 17 stone, I am not easily moved around. I don't sit well in a hoist due to my height, and my carers find transfers difficult, especially from my wheelchair to the bed, the additional height of the air mattress (which I need to lessen the risk of pressure sores) makes getting the height to swing me across difficult. My carers have to manually move my legs to ensure I am properly on the bed.

Another problem is getting dressed and undressed. Due to the delicate condition of my skin, which is breaking down and prone to ulceration, the pulling and tugging of clothing which then gets caught up in the straps of the hoist causes me a lot of discomfort. The spasming that is a major symptom of MS is triggered by the sling straps and makes the transfers even more difficult and uncomfortable.

I find being hoisted undignified, uncomfortable and quite frightening. Having slipped from a sling and endured surgery to mend my left femur, I am very aware of the harm that I could come to during transfers. I find it deeply frustrating to have to rely on others for my every need and have been known to show my frustration on occasions.

Up until 1988, I could use transfer boards and a walking frame together with my wheelchair. Now I am totally dependent on carers. I would be happier if carers were trained in my home to cope with my specific needs, so that I could have input into my care programme. This would help to show me that all my carers understand my case and, most importantly, my needs as an individual."

This book has been written for people who are involved in providing care in the community. By 'community' we mean people's own homes, nursing or residential homes. It is not intended to be used by informal, unpaid carers or relatives since they do not have access to the necessary training and support.

What is 'manual handling'?

This book aims to provide guidance on working safely when supporting people in the community, specifically when they need to move. In providing such guidance, it also aims to reduce to a minimum the accidents and injuries that can happen to all those involved. The term 'manual handling' is widely used. It appears in legislation, regulations, policy and practice documents across a range of different industries, as well as in health and social care settings. 'Manual handling' has also given rise to the phrase 'moving and handling' which is often used, for instance, to describe a particular person's job - the Moving and Handling Adviser.

In the context of this book, 'manual handling' and 'moving and handling' mean the process of transporting or moving another person or an object by hand, or by using the force of the body, for example, by pushing or pulling. We recognise that these terms are impersonal and, in writing a book which focuses on individual people, we have attempted to limit them. However, they are useful terms which carers in the community will encounter and from which we cannot escape. We would urge managers and carers involved in such work to explain what they plan to do in clear terms to the people for whom they are providing care.

In the book, the authors often mention the word '**ergonomic**' - ergonomic approach, ergonomic framework etc. It is important to understand what this means. Ergonomics is basically about ensuring a good 'fit' or 'match' between people, what they do, where they do it and the equipment they use. Each of these elements is important. An ergonomic approach demands that, wherever possible, you should AVOID the need for hazardous manual handling. But where you can't, you must ASSESS the risk of injury and them REDUCE it to the lowest level that is reasonable and possible to put into practice. With work involving manual handling, this means not simply trying to reduce the weight of what has to be moved but looking in turn at all elements of possible risk: what's being done (the task), what's being moved (the load), where it's being done (the working environment), and who's doing it (the individual capability of the person).

How is the guidance organised?

The book is in two broad sections. The first (Chapters 1-5) deals with the important elements of the framework in which carers and care managers operate. Chapter 1 addresses the legislation and regulations which impose responsibility on everyone involved in providing care, including the authority or agency, the care manager and carers themselves. In Chapter 2, we briefly cover the structure and function of the back and look at some of the principles of safer handling.

Chapter 3 introduces the key concept of risk assessment and offers practical advice on what needs to be assessed and how to go about it. In Chapter 4, the importance of training is discussed and we look at what needs to be included in a training programme. Chapter 5 presents some discussion of how best to work with the very wide variety of people that carers will come across each day.

In the second part of the book, we offer practical detail, including advice on equipment (Chapter 6) that can be used both in the home and when going on outings (Chapter 7). In Chapter 8 a comprehensive description of the various techniques which can be used in a range of situations is provided, and this chapter has seventy illustrations showing good practice and warning against the use of unsafe techniques.

A list of References and Further Reading appears at the end of each chapter and at the end of the book we have inserted a list of key organisations with their contact details which readers may find helpful.

Language

Different professions use different words to describe the people they work with - patient, client, service user etc. In this book we have used the words 'Person' or 'People'. With the exception of Chapter 8, we have assumed that the 'Person' being cared for may be either male or female. In Chapter 8 however, we have used the male pronoun (he) when we refer to the Person receiving care, and the female pronoun (she) when referring to the Carer. Although the techniques can be carried out by a male or female carer, we have done this to simplify the description and for clarity and consistency.

The Writing Team

All contributors to this book are people who have direct experience of working in the community or training community-based staff. Not only have they developed considerable expertise through practice and teaching, they have also become champions of the need to follow the principles of safer moving and handling and to think out solutions to moving and handling problems in any working situation, rather than simply following a code. Sound assessment is the key to responding well to a care situation; a range of sound techniques combined with proper training is the key to implementing that response. They also emphasise the fact that self-care is absolutely essential. Personal back care is a 24-hour task which is influenced by work, home, leisure and general lifestyle factors. The importance of a good general level of fitness to support the selection of techniques will also help reduce the toll of back injury.

1 Legislation & Responsibilities
what this means to employer and employee

Ron Steed, Sue Wiltshire, Sally Cassar and Doreen Field.

Background and Principles

Back injuries are not new. The fact that many serious back injuries occur because of manual handling is also not new. The earliest record of back injury is from 1500 BC (the Edwin Smith Egyptian Papyrus). During the Industrial Revolution awareness of the connection between trauma to the spine and back injuries grew. In the 1840s, the term 'railway spine' was used, showing the link between manual work on the railways and back injuries. Eventually, compensation payments were introduced for injured workers. Later on, in the 1930s, orthopaedics emerged as an area of study within medicine. As a result of the increase in knowledge, some of the causes of a 'slipped disc' were identified and the connection between traumatic loading to the spine and back injuries were recognised (Rosen, 1994).

Nearly a third of all workplace accidents reported to the Health and Safety Executive [HSE] involve manual handling. "In the health services that proportion rises to over half... nearly 14,000 manual handling accidents were reported to the HSE and over 60 percent of them involved patient handling" (HSC, 1998). Such statistics are worrying. The concern about health and safety in general, including back injuries, led to the introduction of the Health and Safety at Work etc. Act, 1974 [HSWA] (UK Government, 1974). This Act pulled together many of the disjointed health and safety laws that concentrated on specific industries or work situations. It also required employers and employees to improve the general health and safety of the nation while at work. The HSWA is part of the legal framework of manual handling. The principal objective of this framework of legislation and regulations is to prevent accidents and reduce the number of cases of occupational ill-health. If you have any doubts about responsibilities and accountability then seek legal advice.

The Legal Framework

THE HEALTH AND SAFETY AT WORK ETC. ACT, 1974

This act and its regulations impose a duty on every employer to

'ensure, so far as is reasonably practicable, the health, safety and welfare at work of all his employees'

and

'conduct his undertaking in such a way as to ensure, so far as is reasonably practicable, that persons not in his employment who may be affected thereby are not exposed to risks to their health or safety'.

The HSWA requires:

the **employer** to :

♦ provide safe equipment and systems of work

♦ provide safety in connection with use, storage and transport of loads (including people) and substances hazardous to health

♦ provide understandable information, instruction, training and supervision

♦ maintain safe workplace access and exits

♦ maintain a safe working environment

♦ provide a written health and safety policy statement (if there are 5 or more employees).

the **employee** to:

♦ take reasonable care of his own health and safety and that of other persons at work who may be affected by his actions

♦ co-operate to ensure their own safety and the safety of others at all times

♦ not damage or disable equipment

♦ be willing to receive training.

In essence the HWSA expects employers to manage hazards with the same degree of attention and at the same level of priority as they manage other important aspects of their business, such as the quality of service and allocation of resources. If the employer or employee fails to comply with legislation, they may face criminal or civil proceedings or both. Failure to comply may lead to many more immediate problems as shown in the table below.

Employer Costs	Employee Costs
sickness benefit payments	pain and suffering
overtime payments to other staff	medication and alternative therapy costs
agency replacement costs	
recruitment and induction of replacements	decrease in earnings
bad publicity	restrictions on normal routines (work and social)
decreased staff morale	
investigation by health and safety inspectors	possible legal costs of accident investigation
correcting any faults, defects or damage	
court and legal fees	
compensation costs	
increased insurance premiums	

The HSWA laid the foundations for improved health and safety. It is an enabling Act which allows the Secretary of State to enact other regulations and issue codes of good practice through the Health and Safety Commission [HSC]. However, the HSWA remained vague in some areas and this was a cause of concern to members of the European Community [EC], including the UK. Many European countries bear huge costs in lost productivity annually due to back pain; for the UK the figure is approximately £5 billion every year (CSAG, 1994). Lost productivity, and its associated costs, led to the introduction of a series of EC Directives. In the UK the Directives were introduced and are known as the 'Six Pack of Regulations' (HSE, 1992 (a)-(d) and HSE, 1998 (a)-(b)).

THE SIX PACK OF REGULATIONS

1 **Management of Health and Safety at Work Regulations, 1992 (MHSWR)**
   Sets out broad general duties for improving health and safety, and introduces the requirements for risk assessment and management

2 **Workplace (Health, Safety & Welfare) Regulations, 1992 (HSWR)**
   Sets general requirements to improve the working environment, safety, facilities and housekeeping.

3 **Provision and Use of Work Equipment Regulations, 1998 (PUWER)**
   Sets general duties on employers and lists minimum requirements for work equipment to deal with selected hazards whatever the industry.

4 **Health and Safety (Display Screen Equipment) Regulations, 1992 (DSER)**
   Sets minimum health and safety requirements for work with display screen equipment.

5 **Personal Protective Equipment at Work Regulations, 1992 (PPEWR)**
   Advises on the selection of personal protective equipment, considers different types available and identifies some of the processes and activities that may require it.

6 **Manual Handling Operations Regulations, 1992 (MHOR)**
   Supplements the general duties upon employers concerning the moving of loads and replaces a number of earlier, outdated legal provisions.

These six regulations seek to reinforce and clarify the HSWA and place specific duties on both employer and employee. Here we will consider in more detail the two relevant to this book.

MANAGEMENT OF HEALTH AND SAFETY AT WORK REGULATIONS, 1992 (MHSWR)

The MHSWR are the general regulations requiring the employer, amongst other things, to carry out risk assessments on all tasks considered to be hazardous within the workplace and to reduce risks to a reasonably practicable level. The regulations also require the employer to appoint 'competent persons'. A definition of the main terms used in the regulations is useful:

♦ hazard = potential to cause harm

♦ risk = chance or likelihood of harm occurring and its severity

♦ reasonably practicable - MHSWR reinforces the concept of 'reasonable practicability'. When assessing risks, employers must take appropriate steps to reduce the risk of injury to the lowest level reasonably practicable. These principles of reducing risk are also known as 'SFAIRP' - so far as is reasonably practicable.

The cost (money, time and effort) of introducing changes must be weighed against the likelihood and severity of the risk identified, when the cost is particularly high (1 A11 ER [1949]*). In considering the cost of introducing changes, only the magnitude of the risk is relevant. Assessments and safety changes must be made before, not after an accident/incident.

We can easily define the words 'reasonable' and 'practicable' but the **term 'reasonably practicable'** is more difficult. An illustration might help to clarify this.

* This refers to case law

Illustration

Staff in a nursing home frequently pushed patients to the bathroom on a commode chair with small wheels. They would then lift the person up using a top and tail lift, struggle to the side of the bath tub and lift the person into the bath. They would then assist with bathing the person while maintaining poor postures. When the bath was finished, staff would drain the water, dry the person and top and tail lift the person back onto the commode chair. Staff frequently complained of backache after a morning shift when baths were usually given.

In consultation with a manual handling co-ordinator, the transfer technique (top and tail lift) was identified as involving a very high risk of injury to staff and the person being lifted. At the same time as giving manual handling training to all staff, minor changes were made to the bath tub by raising it sufficiently off the floor to allow a mobile patient hoist to be used. A battery operated mobile hoist was purchased and staff were given training on its use. A wheelchair (already on site) was used to transfer the person to and from the bathroom.

The cost of introducing changes was approximately £2,000. £300 to raise the bath tub; £1,800 for a mobile patient hoist and training provided by the manufacturer. Manual handling training was given to all staff to introduce best techniques and reduce poor postures.

MANUAL HANDLING OPERATIONS REGULATIONS 1992 (MHOR)

MHOR should not be considered in isolation from other relevant legal duties of employers. Again, an understanding of the main terms used is important and these extracts quoted from the guide to the MHOR provide a clear definition:

'manual handling operations mean *any* transporting or supporting of a load (including the lifting, putting down, pushing, pulling, carrying or moving thereof) by hand or bodily force' (Reg. 2(1)).

'A load in this context must be a discrete moveable object. This includes, for example, a human patient receiving medical attention ...' (HSE, 1998).

These Regulations impose specific duties on employers and employees in a clear hierarchy of measures:

the **employer** must:

♦ **avoid** manual handling tasks so far as is reasonably practicable

♦ **assess risk** - if the manual handling task cannot be avoided, the employer must carry out a suitable and sufficient risk assessment of the task and

♦ **eliminate or reduce** - based on the findings of the risk assessment, eliminate or reduce the risk of injury to the lowest level reasonably practicable

♦ **inform** - in addition, HWSA and MHSWR require employers to provide employees with Health and Safety information and training. This should be supplemented as necessary with more specific information and training on manual handling injury risks and prevention, as part of the process of reducing risks as required by MHOR.

the **employee** must:

♦ maintain a reasonable duty of care to self and others

♦ in addition they should co-operate with the employer to help comply with relevant regulations and maintain their health and safety duties. They should inform their employer if tasks are causing problems

♦ make full and proper use of any equipment or system of work provided to them by the employer, in compliance with the regulations (HSE, 1998).

It seems obvious and sensible for a manager to introduce and enforce policies that are 'reasonably practicable'. One of the important policies the manager should introduce that is not required under MHOR but will help to ensure compliance is a *Manual Handling Policy*. This should identify who is accountable for implementing and using the policy (see: Establishing a Policy, page 12). The Manual Handling Policy should also detail the manual handling training required for all staff: methods and standards of manual handling tasks; risk assessments; and methods of monitoring training and risk reduction measures. For coverage of vital aspects of training see Chapter 4.

Responsibilities

A manager must ensure that staff realise that moving and handling is an aspect of all caring activities. Managers can also encourage the application of the principles of safe practice throughout all the activities of daily living. This applies both at work and during leisure time. Care staff must also take responsibility for looking after their own health. A responsible attitude will encourage trust and co-operation. This will help us all to achieve safer practice in the community and a reduction in moving and handling incidents.

A summary of the manager's responsibilities

Managers should create an environment where health and safety is an integral part of the organisation's work practices. This means that, as a manager, you are responsible for making sure that:

1   you translate legal requirements into operational policies and procedures according to the needs of the organisation

2   you consult all relevant staff before new policies and procedures are implemented

3   you distribute new policies and procedures and make sure they are understood before training sessions, so that the trainer and staff are aware of the organisation's requirements. It is, therefore, vital that the timetable for drafting procedures and setting up training is carefully planned

4   you put monitoring arrangements in place following training to observe practice, support staff and offer further training as necessary

5   you review and amend procedures as necessary according to changing organisational needs and/or revised legislation (continuous cycle)

6   you communicate with line managers to ensure they are clear about their responsibilities and the procedures for reporting to senior management or committee members.

To fulfil current legislation and safeguard the health of employees, you have to employ competent people who are skilled in moving and handling. You need to encourage those skilled staff to share their knowledge with other employees and ensure their practice improves continuously throughout the organisation. You could set up a small group of interested people to do this and contribute to the development of the organisation's policies and procedures.

Establishing a policy

The policy must:

♦ fulfil the criteria of the MHOR, 1992 (see page 5 above)

♦ be written clearly so that it is easily understood

♦ be accessible to all staff affected by it

♦ be written in such a way that it can be enforced

♦ be regularly revised and updated at least annually, either by adding further information as a separate appendix or insert, or by reprinting the whole revised document.

The policy must tackle the question of whether to move people manually or with equipment. The introduction of regulations covering manual handling operations, together with the increasing evidence of back injuries resulting from manual handling, has provoked extensive debate during the last few years on whether a '**no lifting**' or a '**minimal lifting**' policy is appropriate. When issues are reduced to catchphrases in this way, they tend to produce division and cause misinterpretation which is unhelpful and can even jeopardise the provision of safe and effective care. For example, 'no lifting' may mistakenly be taken to mean no lifting under any circumstances, but there are clearly instances when lifting is appropriate, such as lifting or moving an object from the floor to avoid tripping over it, or lifting a person's arm to wash them or dress a wound.

On the other hand, 'minimal lifting' is also open to a wide range of interpretations: what is 'minimal' and how is it judged at the moment of providing care? In fact, 'no lifting' means <u>no lifting of all, or most of a person's full body weight</u> except in emergency or life-threatening situations and, spelt out like this, it must be a part of any policy. Common sense suggests that you should make an exception to this when caring for small babies but this should still be clarified in the policy. Even small babies are a possible risk as there are many other factors aside from their weight which may compromise safe handling; for example, the capability of the person caring for the baby, difficult environmental conditions, or if the baby has any disability.

It is best to debate these issue within your organisation, and whether an individual or organisation decides on a 'no lifting' or the 'minimal lifting' policy is, in the end, unimportant. The top priority is to establish a policy that is clear and unambiguous, practical and enforceable. If the policy is well written, it will not be misinterpreted. It is also of prime importance that the policy exists within a philosophical framework that promotes the independence and dignity of the person receiving care, at the same time as protecting the health and well-being of those who provide it.

WRITING THE POLICY

1. Policy statement

When deciding how to write a policy you might consider issuing a brief 'Policy Statement'. This should help to establish the general principles of health and safety relating to moving and handling within the organisation. You could do this by means of a short statement easily read by everyone. Social Services Departments should have a Moving and Handling Policy for their employees. Although this may not be suitable in its entirety for the particular organisation in which you are involved, you may be able to adapt it to suit the needs of your staff and the people to whom they provide care.

2. Staff accountability

In the second part of the policy, you should concentrate on those key members of staff who will be accountable for its implementation. You need to state their responsibilities clearly to ensure each person knows exactly what is expected of them. These key members of staff should include some or all of the following:

- Senior managers - Chief Executive, Director etc.
- Moving and Handling Adviser
- Heads of Service
- Departmental Management Team
- Departmental Safety Co-ordinator
- Training Manager
- Care Managers
- Care Staff
- Volunteers
- Agency Employees
- Outside Contractors.

3. Procedures

Moving and handling procedures should form the third part of the policy. You should address the following issues:

♦ general risk assessment

♦ individual risk assessment

♦ principles of safer practice

♦ training procedures

♦ a method of monitoring the effectiveness of the policy.

You can get guidance for writing a safety policy statement from the Health and Safety Executive (HSC, 1993).

Training

Providing training is a central responsibility of management and is discussed in detail in Chapter 4. The principles of safer practice should form the basis of a training programme, and you should encourage carers to use common sense and tact in a moving and handling situation rather than applying a rigid set of rules. All managers should be familiar with these basic principles, as should each member of staff. The content of basic training courses should include all those aspects considered essential to raise awareness among the participants.

Training programmes should also incorporate the aims and targets for the organisation.

AIMS

The aims should state the following:

1 An agreed amount of time is allocated.

2 The quality of training should be to a recognised standard as agreed by professional bodies (e.g. The Royal College of Nursing, The Chartered Society of Physiotherapists). It should cover those aspects considered by the organisation as essential to meet the needs of the people requiring care.

3 The training should be available to all existing staff involved in moving and handling people and to all new members of staff within a specified time limit (ideally before commencing work in people's homes).

4 All managers of staff who move people should receive training in risk assessment.

5 All staff identified as at risk of injury as a result of moving and handling activities should receive suitable training.

TARGETS

The targets should state the following:

1 Managers to be provided with names of staff who have attended training in order to monitor attendance.

2 Sufficient courses to be provided to meet the aims of the organisation.

3 Refresher training courses to be provided for staff on an annual basis.

Management issues within the Purchaser-Provider relationship

LEGAL OBLIGATIONS

The service purchaser and the service provider must each fulfil certain obligations. The National Health Service and Community Care Act, 1990 requires local authorities to separate purchasing and provider activities.

Aim

To ensure the assessment of care (purchasing) is seen as independent from the provider activity and determined by the needs of the people requiring care.

Objectives

♦ Purchasers must ensure that the care agencies they use meet the specified standards of the organisation before purchasing care.

♦ Service providers must guarantee they are competent to meet the needs of the purchaser.

♦ Service providers must ensure that there are suitable care staff who are sufficiently trained in all aspects of care, including carrying out basic moving and handling risk assessment and safe practice.

In order to guarantee that approved agencies meet local specified criteria, the agencies should be regularly reviewed by the purchasers. These approved agencies can be local authorities or from the independent sector and it is possible, therefore, that a Person may receive services from more than one agency. Liaison between all providers via the Care Manager is essential in order to ensure continuity of care.

Private organisations which do not contract with the local authority should be aware of the need to liaise directly with other professionals as necessary.

COMMUNICATION ISSUES

Communication between Social Services providers and purchasers and all agencies on their approved list is essential. Lines of communication should be clear so that all parties can be well informed. Written care plans and appropriate risk assessments should be available for all staff involved in the care of any Person in the community (see Chapter 3: Assessing Risks). These care plans should include recommendations for safer moving of the person.

SUPPORT FOR FRONT LINE CARE STAFF

A Moving and Handling Adviser should be provided by the care organisations to directly support their staff when caring for particular People in their own homes. These specialist workers enhance the support afforded to the Person, to any informal carers and to the paid staff. The ability to teach in the Person's home, and also teach groups of staff from all agencies involved in the care of a particular Person, can be beneficial to all concerned (see Chapter 4: Training). If necessary, to ensure safe practice takes place, the Moving and Handling Adviser can produce detailed moving and handling care plans. These should be accessible to all concerned with the care of the Person. The individual member of staff responsible for the Person's needs should carry out basic risk assessment when caring for the Person.

In addition, senior care assistants should be able to support staff, particularly new recruits, in safer moving and handling practice, and encourage them to alert their manager and the Moving and Handling Adviser of potential risks. In this way risk can be minimised so accidents do not occur.

OTHER HEALTH PROFESSIONALS

A holistic approach to moving and handling is essential in the community. The ideals of the holistic, or whole approach, can be applied to the group of people involved in maintaining the Person's health and well-being and also to the care or treatment actually given.

People involved may include the Person and their family, general practitioner, district nurse, occupational therapist, physiotherapist, paid care staff and a specialised Moving and Handling Adviser. All these people have a specific role; their care and practice should enable them to work together to achieve a quality service for the Person.

An example may help to clarify the approach and its benefits.

Illustration

A Person suffering from periodic acute spasms knocks delicate skin during an attack, causing a severe graze or bruise. The doctor and district nurse are alerted by care staff to the situation. The doctor prescribes suitable medication to control the attacks and dressings to ensure healing takes place. Although the Person has been able to walk and get to bed with assistance prior to the attack, the district nurse advises rest temporarily. The Moving and Handling Adviser visits and assists the Person, care staff and family to maintain safer moving and handling practice, providing equipment if appropriate. If necessary, the physiotherapist can be alerted by the general practitioner in order to assist with rehabilitation once healing has occurred. The positive aspects of this approach promote high standards of care and may result in a speedier recovery for the Person and a safer environment for all concerned.

Your responsibilities as a carer

Your responsibilities as a carer are to implement good practice within the framework provided by your manager.

◆ To provide the best and safest quality of care possible under the given circumstances. By using safer moving techniques the quality of care will be enhanced.

◆ To use the equipment and systems of work (handling techniques) provided by the employer and outlined in the local policy.

◆ To be sensitive and diplomatic at all times and most especially when working in a Person's own home.

◆ To discuss with each Person their fears and expectations as well as their preferences about how they are moved and cared for.

◆ To discuss any ideas for any changes to the home or for the use of any specialised equipment etc. so that the Person has time to understand and accept them.

◆ To recognise that, based upon risk assessment, some People will be unable either to physically transfer or move by themselves, or will be able to do so only with assistance from a carer. In this situation you, the carer, must reduce the risks for both the Person and yourself by using safer moving techniques and by introducing appropriate equipment. You must also recognise that some People may say they can move safely by themselves when their physical condition means that they cannot. To allow them to continue to attempt self-powered movement, or to participate in such physical transfers, would be hazardous and should not be done.

♦ To recognise that there are many People who are capable of carrying out some or many activities of daily life without assistance. At times, by encouraging self-help, there will be benefits for the Person and the carer. The Person retains as much dignity and control of their environment as is possible and the risks of injury associated with manual handling and moving are decreased.

♦ To undertake regular reassessment. Regular reassessment is essential, especially as an Person's ability to assist the carer and contribute to any move can vary. For example, conditions such as multiple sclerosis may result in periods of time when a Person is totally dependent and other periods of time when they are able to move themselves with very little support or assistance. It is vital to encourage independence and secure the Person's maximum participation in the transfers; this helps to maintain dignity, morale and strength.

♦ To be aware that there are potential dangers in enabling a Person to assist the carer in a move, but at the same time to ensure that the person is not deprived of the ability to participate. Plan to minimise risks.

♦ To provide feedback and regular liaison are key responsibilities of the carer, especially if there is a need to deviate from the care plan. There may be a number of agencies providing care for the same Person and they all need to communicate so that care is consistent. It is also important to liaise with other carers or therapists who may be involved in supporting the Person. This will ensure that a handling programme is written which allows a safe system of work at all times. If all parties agree on the care plan, then conflict between what a carer expects to do and what the Person expects them to do can be avoided. This prevents carers taking risks or being put at risk by feeling obliged to carry out a task in an unsafe way because another carer has done so previously.

♦ To be conscious of the limitations of your skills and knowledge and that of other carers. Work within these limitations and do not take unnecessary risks.

REFERENCES

1 A11 ER [1949]. Edwards v. National Coal Board [1949]. 1 All ER 743.

Clinical Standards Advisory Group (CSAG), (1994). Back Pain: Report of CSAG, Committee on Back Pain. HMSO, London.

HSC, (1993). Leaflet 4/86, revised 1993. Writing a Safety Policy Statement: Advice to Employers HMSO, London.

HSC, (1998). Manual Handling in the Health Services, Second Edition. HMSO, London.

HSE, (1992 (a)). Guidance on Management of Health and Safety Regulations. HMSO, London.

HSE, (1992 (b)). Guidance on Workplace (Health Safety and Welfare) Regulations. HMSO, London.

HSE, (1992 (c)). Guidance on Health and Safety (Display Screen Equipment) Regulations. HMSO, London.

HSE, (1992 (d)). Guidance on Personal Protective Equipment at Work Regulations. HMSO, London.

HSE, (1998 (a)). Guidance on Manual Handling Operations Regulations. HMSO, London.

HSE, (1998 (b)). Guidance on Provision and Use of Work Equipment Regulations. HMSO, London.

Rosen, M., (1994). Back Pain, Report of a Clinical Standards Advisory Group Committee on Back Pain: 7-8. HMSO, London.

UK Government, (1974). Health and Safety at Work etc. Act. HMSO, London.

FURTHER READING

Chartered Society of Physiotherapists, (1995). Standards of Physiotherapy Practice for Trainers in Moving and Handling. Chartered Society of Physiotherapists, London.

Chartered Society of Physiotherapists, (1998). Moving and Handling for Chartered Physiotherapists. Chartered Society of Physiotherapists, London.

Commission of European Communities (CEC), (1990). Council Directive of 29 May, 1990 (90/269/EEC) on the minimum health and safety requirements for the manual handling of loads where there is a risk particularly of back injury to workers (Fourth Individual Directive within the meaning of Article 16 (1) of Directive 89/391/EEC). Official Journal of the European Communities, No L156/9-12, Brussels.

DfEE, (1996). The Disability Discrimination Act Definition of Disability: Disability on the Agenda. DfEE, London.

Dept. of Employment, (1993). Code of Good Practice on the Employment of Disabled People. HMSO, London.

HSC, (1997). Management of Health and Safety in the Health Services. HSE Books, London.

HSE, (1994). A Pain in your Workplace? Ergonomic Problems and Solutions. HSE Books, London.

HSE, (1994). Five Steps to Successful Health and Safety Management. IND(G) 132L. HSE Books, London.

HSE, (1994). Manual Handling Solutions You Can Handle. HS(G) 115, HSE Books, London.

HSE, (1995). Health Risk Management: A Practical Guide for Managers in Small and Medium-sized Enterprises. HS(G) 137. HSE Books, London.

National Back Pain Association, (1998). The Guide to the Handling of Patients, Fourth Edition. National Back Pain Association in collaboration with the Royal College of Nursing, London.

Royal College of Nursing, (1996). Introducing a Safer Patient Handling Policy. RCN, London.

UK Government, (1995). Disability Discrimination Act. HMSO, London.

2 **Principles of safer handling**

Joyce Cheney

Your Back

Your back is an ingenious feat of engineering. You need to treat it with care because it is one of the most important parts of the body. A healthy back is important in allowing you to get the most out of life. Your back lets you walk, stand, lift, bend, work, play and sleep; it is also one of the parts of the body most prone to injury. It only has to be injured once and you could be troubled with a back problem for the rest of your life. Your spine is in use 24 hours a day - even when you are asleep.

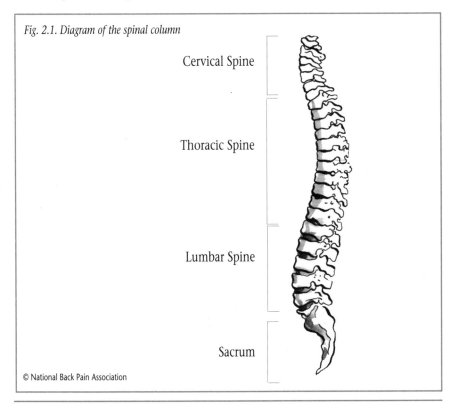

Fig. 2.1. Diagram of the spinal column

Cervical Spine

Thoracic Spine

Lumbar Spine

Sacrum

STRUCTURE AND FUNCTION

Your spine is a complex structure of bones (the vertebrae) which are stacked one on top of the other. They work together with the muscles, tendons and ligaments to provide an impressive range of movements, as well as supporting your body. The spine also provides protection for the spinal cord. The vertebrae are separated by cushions called inter-vertebral discs, which allow the spine to move while acting as shock absorbers. The disc is made up of strong fibrous outer layers encasing a soft central area, which changes shape when you move. The spine is not perfectly straight (Fig. 2.1) but has natural curves which support your weight and absorb stress. If you move when these natural curves are not present, the stress on the spine increases leading to back injuries, if there is too much of the wrong kind of movement over a period of time. This is due to additional pressures and stress on the discs, joints and ligaments. The lower region of the back is the most vulnerable part since it bears the weight of the trunk of your body as well as the weight of any load you carry.

FORCES ON THE SPINE

For your spine to work efficiently, it is essential that your joints are in a neutral position (Fig. 2.2a) with the natural curves present, since this requires minimum forces from muscles acting on joints and discs. When you bend your trunk forwards (Fig. 2.2b and 2.2c), the forces acting on your spine to maintain the position are increased. These forces become greater with further bending; adding a weight, such as groceries, a child or (worse still) an adult, increases them further.

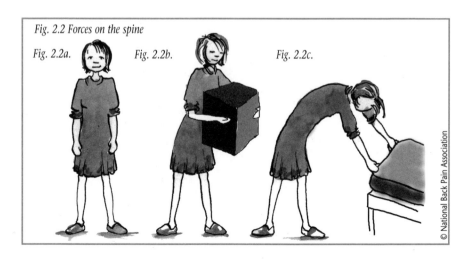

Fig. 2.2 Forces on the spine

Fig. 2.2a. *Fig. 2.2b.* *Fig. 2.2c.*

© National Back Pain Association

The squeezing (compression)* and shearing* effects from the extra forces have a cumulative effect on the joints, ligaments and discs, leading to damage. In addition to keeping a good posture, it is very important that you keep any load close to your body since outstretched arms put extra pressure on the trunk, low back and shoulders, increasing the force required to maintain your position. Twisted postures (Fig. 2.2c) and sudden movements can cause undesirable stress to the discs, joints and soft tissues of the spine.

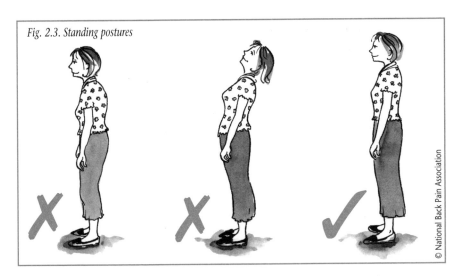

Fig. 2.3. Standing postures

© National Back Pain Association

CAUSES OF LOW BACK PAIN

There are many causes of low back pain, most of which we can actually influence.

♦ Poor posture (Fig. 2.3) - slouching, rounded shoulders, raised arms, twisted spine, sitting or standing slightly bent over frequently or for long periods can result in cumulative strain. It is important to avoid maintaining any posture or movement for a long period of time. Maintaining fixed postures over time is often referred to as adopting static postures.

♦ Degeneration - the normal ageing process produces wear and tear in all the weightbearing joints including the spine. The amount of wear and tear will vary from one person to the next and may be accelerated by other factors such as the additional stresses placed on the spine by excess weight.

♦ Lack of exercise - leads to weak abdominal and back muscles, affects your posture and can, therefore, lead to back pain.

*Compression: see Glossary *Shearing: see Glossary

- Poor ergonomic assessment - failure to consider all aspects including the load, the task, the Person and the working environment (see Chapter 3: Assessing Risks).

- Traumatic injury caused by sudden violent stresses applied to the spine.

Principles of safer handling

1. Avoid manual lifting where possible.

2. Assess what needs to be done.

3. Assess the situation, the person or object to be moved.

4. Use equipment whenever possible to reduce the risk of injury.

5. Know your limitations.

6. Prepare the area - space, position of furniture etc.

7. Communicate with all team members including the person who is being moved.

8. Get into position:

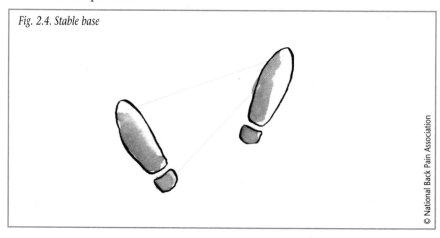

Fig. 2.4. Stable base

© National Back Pain Association

- your feet apart for a wide, stable base (comfortable, non-slip shoes); place your leading foot in the direction of travel (Fig. 2.4)

- your spine in position with natural curves present

- avoid twisting

- keep close to the load

- have your knees and hips bent

  Bent knees allow you to reach lower while maintaining your natural spinal curves. This also allows you to support the load closer to your body. This approach reduces the load on all structures of your body, including the back and shoulders.

- keep a good hold on the load

- have your elbows tucked in

- keep your abdominal muscles tight.

9. Perform the move:

- raise your head as you move, keep shoulders relaxed

- smooth movement.

10. Evaluate the move. Did it go well? If not, why not? What would make it easier or safer?

Useful tips for a healthy back

Most back pain is avoidable - but only you can prevent it.

POSTURE:

- Try to maintain an upright posture at all times; avoid hunching your shoulders - walk tall.

- Make sure your back is in position with the natural curves present when moving loads or working at low levels.

- Use your strong thigh and buttock muscles so you don't have to bend your back.

- Muscles take a long time to recover if they become exhausted, so it is important to rest between tasks.

WEIGHT:

- It is important to control your weight as excess weight exerts a constant forward pull on the low back due to the bulk of the abdomen. The final outcome is wear and tear on the joints - and possible pain.

BED:

♦ Since you spend so much time in bed, it is important to have a mattress that supports your back.

CAR:

♦ Ensure your car seat is firm and supports the natural curves of your back. If your car seat gives you little or no support, you could try a cushion, a rolled towel or one of the many manufactured supports.

HOME/WORK:

♦ You should try to avoid bending over work surfaces; perhaps sitting or kneeling is an option e.g. when making the beds or cleaning the bath.

♦ Keep objects that you use frequently in cupboards or on shelves that you can reach without overstretching. If you have to reach into high cupboards, it is safer to use steps rather than a chair.

LOAD MOVING:

♦ Always ask yourself: "Does it have to be moved?" If it does, then apply the principles above. Do not carry a heavy load in one hand; try to split the load and carry equal amounts on both sides. If you are concerned about moving a person in your care you should talk to your manager.

KEEP FIT AND FLEXIBLE:

♦ It has been shown that good fitness levels are significant in preventing low back pain and reducing stress levels. Swimming and brisk walking are both excellent forms of exercise. If you exercise regularly, it will help fitness; 3 times a week for 20 to 30 minutes is a good guide. A selection of gentle mobility and flexibility exercises is shown below. These should not cause pain, but if you do experience pain you should stop and seek advice.

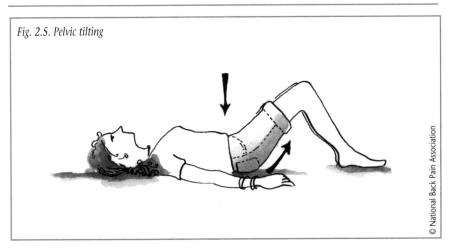

Fig. 2.5. Pelvic tilting

© National Back Pain Association

Pelvic tilting (Fig. 2.5)

Lie with both knees bent, feet on the floor, and your hands flat on the floor under your back at just below waist level. Try to flatten your back to the floor by tilting your pelvis up and tightening your abdominal muscles. Hold for a count of 20 (while breathing normally), then release. Repeat 10 times.

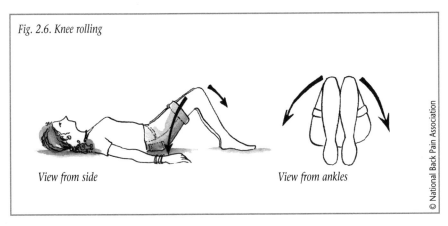

Fig. 2.6. Knee rolling

View from side

View from ankles

© National Back Pain Association

Knee rolling

Lying as above, gently roll your knees from side to side as far as you comfortably can. Repeat 10 times.

Fig. 2.7. Humping and hollowing

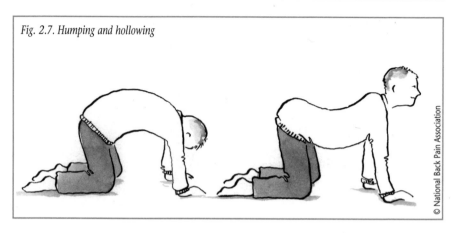

Humping and hollowing (Fig. 2.7)

Starting in position on all fours, hump and hollow your back in an easy gentle movement. Raise your head as you hollow your back, and lower your head as you hump your back. Repeat 5 - 10 times.

3 **Assessing Risks**

Julian Pearce and Sally Cassar

The Purpose of Risk Assessment

We undertake risk assessment to identify problem areas so that prevention measures can be put in place to make a situation as safe as possible for all concerned. The mere mention of the issue of risk assessment makes many people nervous and causes them to question their ability. This is a pity because risk assessment is something that everyone does every day of their life, often without realising it.

Imagine you are in your car at a T junction wanting to turn right. You look left, it's clear; you look right and there is a milk float 400 metres away. In that moment you perform a risk assessment. There is a hazard coming towards you (the milk float), but you estimate that the risk of it hitting you is minimal, so you pull across the road and head on your way.

HAZARD OR RISK?

There are two words used in that description that are often confused: Hazard and Risk. Before we go any further we will consider what they mean because they are key words in the process of risk assessment.

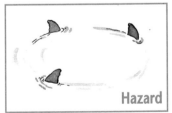
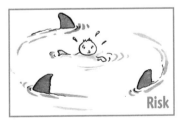

(Reproduced with kind permission of the HSE)

Hazard:

Anything with the potential to cause harm (e.g. a faulty electrical item, a heavy unstable load, an electrical appliance lead running across a floor).

Risk:

The chance that harm will occur and its severity.

Risk can be categorised as:

> **Low** - Where harm is possible but unlikely and of low consequence
>
> **Medium** - Where harm is likely to occur and the injury is significant
>
> **High** - Where harm is very likely to occur and the injury would be major.

Eliminating high risk activities

If you identify a high risk activity, then you MUST take action immediately to reduce the level of risk. You may have to remove someone temporarily into a different type of care while risk reduction is implemented. A manager should not knowingly send a carer to a high risk situation.

Reducing risks

However, you must also give priority to medium and low risks. Sometimes you cannot eliminate risk factors, but you can manage to reduce the risk to a more acceptable level. For example, People with severe rheumatoid arthritis often have particular pain and stiffness on waking. Carers who need to provide help with washing, dressing and assisting such a Person onto a commode may find that they can do these tasks more safely and comfortably later in the morning after an analgesic has taken effect and, hence, they may adapt their care plan accordingly.

Managing the Risks

AN EXAMPLE

Now let's apply the terms hazard and risk to a care situation where we need a risk assessment. As a manager you are responsible for the delivery of care to an elderly lady who is confined to bed upstairs in the house she shares with her husband. You and your staff have had concerns about the safety of the house for some time. The floor boards seem rotten and you have been trying to persuade the couple to move to more suitable accommodation. Today, when a member of your team was climbing the stairs, one stair gave way under her weight.

Using the terms we defined, what is the **hazard** and what is the **risk**? How would you, as a manager, manage that risk? You will have recognised that the condition of the stair, and therefore the entire flooring, is a hazard, and that the chances of that hazard affecting your staff (the risk) is high. You will, therefore, act quickly to make sure that nobody is exposed to the risk any longer than is absolutely necessary. As a manager you need to recognise the risk and take the necessary action to minimise the chance of anyone being injured. This, then, is the essence of risk assessment or, as many people prefer to call it, risk management.

LOCAL POLICY

Local policies within Local Authorities and Area Health Authorities vary and it may not be the role of the care manager to carry out the full Manual Handling Risk Assessment. It is vital, however, that the care manager identifies the need for a full Moving and Handling Assessment of Risk so that the carer has the maximum possible information before visiting the Person for the first time. This may mean that a senior carer, trained and competent in risk assessment, needs to visit the Person before carers are sent in. It is helpful if whoever carries out the risk assessment is familiar with the limitations and abilities of the team who will provide the care.

A major area of concern is when a Person is discharged into the community from hospital. It is essential that an assessment of moving and handling needs is done **prior** to discharge in conjunction with those who will be providing the continuing care. The care manager must insist that either a home visit takes place or, if this is not possible, a safe system is in place following the assessment. A home visit and liaison between care providers is the best way to ensure that safe systems of work are in place at the moment of discharge. Carers should not be confronted with a situation where they have to care for a person without the appropriate equipment or systems of work to carry out the tasks safely.

Three types of assessment

In the 'rotten floor board' scenario you would not question that there was a risk; you would be certain. With moving and handling we often need to be convinced there is a real risk. Why? For many years the risks associated with moving and handling were seen as simply a part of the job - you got on with it; it was expected. Now, however, managers have an unquestionable duty to make sure they undertake risk assessments, not only on the working environments of staff but also in relation to the People they care for. A good approach to managing risk in the caring world involves a three-part process:

- a general risk assessment
- a Moving and Handling Care Plan or Personal Handling Profile
- a generic risk assessment.

The general assessment

The assessor needs to know what can or may cause an injury and how likely it is that it will occur. The booklet 'Manual Handling - Guidance on Regulations' (HSE, 1998) is useful in this respect. It clearly divides risk assessment into four sections which can easily be remembered by using the word LITE.

L   Load - the Person or object to be moved - you need to consider the weight, size etc.

I   Individual - who is providing the care? Can this be safely managed by each member of staff?

T   Task - what has to be done, how and when? Normally this will involve moving a Person in some way.

E   Environment - where is the Person being cared for? Is there enough space? Is the bed too low?

The aim is to identify the hazards or risks within these areas and, in this way, to be aware of the whole picture. These sections help form the basis of an ergonomic assessment, looking at the worker in relation to the environment, the task and the work system. It may be useful for managers to seek advice and information from the Person and from others who have been involved, such as nurses, doctors, therapists, family members and friends.

You can use standardised forms. The form below, with a couple of minor changes in order, has been published by the Health and Safety Executive (HSE, 1998) and acts as a checklist which allows you to work through the four key areas, asking specific questions to prompt your thought processes.

Having determined how much of a risk is posed, you then need to detail what you will do about it - in the words of the form, what remedial action you need to take. This may involve moving furniture or providing a hospital bed and commode; you will also need to detail carefully how any moving of the Person will be performed. This is where the Personal Handling Profile comes in (see below, page 35).

Manual Handling of Loads
EXAMPLE OF AN ASSESSMENT CHECKLIST

SUMMARY OF ASSESSMENT	
Operations covered by this assessment:	Overall priority for remedial action: Nil/Low/Med/High* Remedial action to be taken:
Locations:	Date by which action is to be taken:
Personnel involved:	Date for reassessment:
Date of assessment:	Assessor's name:
	Signature:

*circle as appropriate

Section A - Preliminary:

QI Do the operations involve a significant risk of injury?   Yes/No
If 'Yes' go to Q2. If 'No' the assessment need go no further.
If in doubt answer 'Yes'. You may find the guidelines in Appendix 1 (HSE, 1998) helpful.

Q2 Can the operations be avoided / mechanised / automated at reasonable cost?   Yes/No
If 'No' go to Q3. If 'Yes' proceed and then check that the result is satisfactory.

Q3 Are the operations clearly within the guidelines in Appendix 1(HSE, 1998) ?   Yes/No
If 'No' go to Section B. If 'Yes' you may go straight to Section C if you wish.

Section B - More detailed assessment, where necessary:

Questions to consider: (If the answer to a question is 'Yes' place a tick against it and then consider the level of risk)			Level of risk (Tick as appropriate)			Possible remedial action: (Make rough notes in this column in preparation for completing Section D)
The **TASKS** - do they involve:	Yes	No	Low	Med	High	
holding loads away from the trunk?						
twisting?						
stooping?						
reaching upwards?						
large vertical movement?						
long carrying distances?						
strenuous pushing or pulling?						
unpredictable movement of loads?						
repetitive handling?						
insufficient rest or recovery?						
a workrate imposed by a process?						

The **TASKS** - do they involve:	Yes	No	Low	Med	High	
INDIVIDUAL capability - does the job: require unusual capability? hazard those with a health problem? hazard those who are pregnant? call for special information/training?						
The **LOADS** - are they: heavy? bulky/unwieldy? difficult to grasp? unstable/unpredictable? intrinsically harmful (eg sharp/hot)?						
The working **ENVIRONMENT** - are there: constraints on posture? poor floors? tripping/slipping hazards? variations in levels (e.g. steps)? hot/cold/humid conditions? strong air movements? poor lighting conditions? a workrate imposed by a process?						
Other factors Is movement or posture hindered by clothing or personal protective equipment?						

Deciding the level of risk will inevitably call for judgement. The guidelines in Appendix 1 (HSE, 1998) may provide a useful yardstick.

When you have completed Section B go to Section C.

Section C - Overall assessment of risk:

Q What is your overall assessment of the risk of injury?   Insignificant / Low / Med / High*
If not 'Insignificant' go to Section D. If 'Insignificant' the assessment need go no further.

Section D - Remedial action:

Q What remedial steps should be taken, in order of priority?

i. _____ iv. _____

ii. _____ v. _____

iii. _____

and finally:

- complete the SUMMARY above
- compare it with your other manual handling assessments
- decide your priorities for action
- TAKE ACTION................. AND CHECK THAT IT HAS THE DESIRED EFFECT.

Personal Handling Profile

Care planning must be systematic. Many people are already familiar with the concept of documenting moving and handling information in a Moving and Handling Care Plan or Personal Handling Profile (PHP). There must be one for every Person who needs to be moved (HSE, 1998). The basic idea is to detail the moving situations in which 'handling' is needed and then outline exactly what type of 'handling' is required. The classic response to what type of handling is needed is 'with two', which really tells us nothing other than that two carers are needed. This could mean two carers and a mobile sling hoist with a medium quick-fit sling (legs crossed); it could mean two carers with a handling belt assisting the Person to stand; or it could mean two carers are needed to give verbal instructions and support while the Person transfers themselves using a sliding board. We must retain an overview of the hazards/risk factors to which we are exposed. The following checklist for assessing risks, again based on the 'LITE' concept, may be helpful.

RISK FACTOR CHECKLIST (see Personal Handling Profile (page 41))

The LOAD - the Person or object to be moved

Remember - if you were the Person being moved, what would you want your carers to be aware of?

- weight, size, shape, abnormalities and restricted movements
- vulnerable areas, skin, bones, specific joints, sores, wounds etc.
- weakness, paralysis and impaired muscle tone
- balance, stability, ability to weightbear and for how long and with what support
- coordination
- hypersensitive areas or loss of sensation or awareness of body parts
- ability to step and walk and with what support
- frequency or history of dizzy spells or falling
- any aids used
- personal likes and dislikes
- medical conditions which may affect safety to Person or carer

- ability to understand, follow instructions, feedback and communicate
- sight, hearing and speech
- cultural considerations, modesty, fear
- memory and confusion
- continence
- contagious illness
- attachments, splints, braces, catheters, stoma bags drips, drains etc.

It is important to be precise with information. For example, if the Person has pain, document where the pain site is; if a Person can weightbear, say for how long and whether any support is needed and if so from what or by whom?

If the load is an inanimate object additional questions should be answered:

- Can the object be easily gripped?
- Can the object be broken down into smaller, lighter parts?
- How stable is it?
- What are its contents?
- Is it toxic or hazardous?
- Is it affected by other regulations (e.g. COSHH (Control of Substances Hazardous to Health))?
- Is it attached to anything?
- Is it bulky or unwieldy?

Loads which are similar can be assessed on a generic basis but all sections of LITE must be taken into account. To avoid unnecessary assessment, it may be useful to refer to Appendix 1 of Manual Handling - Guidance on Regulations (HSE, 1998) as this gives guidance on when an assessment may be required.

The INDIVIDUAL - Who is providing the care

Managers must look for factors in their staff which may affect how safely they work. These may include:

- weight, size and strength of carers in relation to the Person, or to each other when working in a team

- vulnerabilities in carers e.g. pregnancy, previous injury, recent illness, stress
- level of knowledge, skills and recent relevant training
- staff attitude towards local policy and the use of equipment (see Chapter 1: Legislation and Responsibilities and Chapter 6: Equipment)
- whether staff are from different agencies or employers who may have a different approach (see Chapter 1: Legislation and Responsibilities)
- expectations
- willingness to follow instructions
- whether staff are in a hurry
- current workload and time of day.

It is vital that appropriate carers with necessary skills and attributes are matched to the Person who needs care and support. For example, it is futile and could be dangerous to have a carer of short stature help a very tall man to stand. Managers must be prepared to assess situations constantly, identify risks and put in risk reduction measures as necessary.

Carers must not be put at risk by feeling expected to do a task with which they are unhappy. Therapists aiming to optimise the rehabilitation potential of People they are treating may have taught techniques that are inappropriate for carers to undertake. There must be feedback between managers, carers and all involved to ensure consistency of care and to make sure that carers are not putting themselves at risk by trying to conform to the wishes of another person.

Example

A carer working with a heavy man who had recently had a stroke was prepared to manually assist using an unsafe bearhug transfer because his wife was worried that the hoist would damage the paintwork in the house. Because one carer had been persuaded to use this unsafe technique, the wife put pressure on all carers to do the same. Eventually there was an injury. The hoist should have been used by all carers.

The TASK - What has to be done and what factors are involved

Questions regarding the task and what it may involve will help identify specific risk factors which can then be dealt with by the manager prior to giving care.

- Is the task necessary?

- How much is the Person contributing to the move?

- Can the task be mechanised or automated, and if so are there additional hazards?

- Is the task repetitive?

- How many staff are required?

- What equipment is required and is it accessible?

- What postures are being adopted by carers?

- Is there lifting or taking significant amounts of weight?

- How long will the task take?

- Is there a need to stoop, reach, twist or hold a load away from the body? Is there a need to maintain an awkward posture?

- Can manual handling be avoided altogether?

- Is this one single task or is this one of many tasks?

- How much is the Person able to contribute to the manoeuvre?

For example, shaving a severely disabled man in his wheelchair will involve standing and stooping for long periods. The same man could be shaved while sitting in his bath hoist chair when in a raised position, thus reducing the degree of forward stooping by the carer. The risk of back injury through stooping while holding a load away from the body can also be reduced. For example, to assist someone to a sitting position from lying on a low soft bed, you can use a mattress inclinator or mechanical pillow lifter (see Chapter 6: Equipment).

The ENVIRONMENT - where the Person is being cared for

Delivering care in the community presents a number of environmental risks. It is vital that managers, carers and People needing support work together to make the environment as safe as possible. There is often a need for diplomacy and sensitivity to persuade People to accept equipment or changes in their surroundings. The benefits must be clearly explained. It is essential that equipment and environment are compatible (see Chapter 5: The Person and the Environment). Again, questions help to identify potential problems.

- Is there a lack of space?

- What height are the working surface levels? Are there low beds, chairs? Are they fixed?

- Is there clutter?
- Are there loose rugs, carpets, worn or unstable flooring?
- Are there any slippery floors?
- Are there steps, stairs or slopes?
- Are there secure grab rails and are they of use?
- Are there other family members? Pets?
- What are the general levels of ventilation, heating, lighting and extremes of temperature? Can they affect safety?
- Are there any electrical, gas or chemical hazards?
- Are there any other hazards?

For example, if family members insist that all bars of a fire are switched on in a poorly ventilated bathroom to prevent the Person becoming cold, the carers themselves may be overcome with heat.

All four areas of the assessment (LITE) are interdependent and should be conducted within an ergonomic framework (RCN, 1996).

Care in the Community - the current ethos

It is important to remember that the current ethos underpinning care in the community is to allow individual choice. There may be times when a Person wishes to take risks. Taking risks is a part of normal life and managers and staff will be helped to make an appropriate judgment by having a clear framework setting out the issues. Most organisations which provide care services will have a list of principles and values for service delivery. Often one such value is that the Person should have the 'right' to take risks. This right may at times be difficult to protect, especially if it endangers someone else. Good communication between the Person, their relatives and the carers involved can help to resolve situations of conflict. It is vital that the care manager coordinates any changes to the care plan so that risk is minimised.

> **Example**
>
> An elderly man used to be transferred by standing from wheelchair to bed has recently deteriorated in physical ability and now needs a mobile sling hoist. He has reluctantly accepted the hoist is coming, but unfortunately, six days before the hoist arrived, the bed was raised and the room reorganised. This made it extremely difficult to continue safely with transferring by standing, which became significantly more hazardous during the six days.

Assessments often result in recommendations for equipment and for changes within the home to facilitate care. If the Person refuses to accept these changes, then there will be no safe system of work in place. If all negotiations fail between managers and the Person then you may need to limit care to the low risk activities until the recommendations are implemented.

DOCUMENTATION

It is essential to have a clearly identifiable personal handling profile (PHP) for all carers to access (see below, page 41). Where more than one agency is involved, it is useful to have a copy in the Person's home. The form should identify the risks or problems involved with moving the Person and give clear guidelines on methods to reduce risks to all parties. This may raise concerns regarding confidentiality, especially if several carers from several different agencies are involved with a Person. It is important that all carers have adequate information so that risks are reduced; however, there may be a medical condition which the Person would prefer to keep confidential. Managers must be aware of how such a condition might affect a carer and whether it implies any additional risk when providing care to the Person. There may be local policies on confidentiality which determine how much information a carer has available in writing on the PHP. It is important that these concerns are addressed and that the Person's permission is sought so that any information which may affect risk is known to all carers.

REASSESSMENT

It is vital that there is someone to contact if problems arise, and that there is ongoing reassessment and monitoring of any moving and handling situation. Carers must be aware that they need to contact their managers to request a reassessment when there is a change in a Person's condition - for better or for worse. Carers are the link in the chain and it is essential that they are encouraged and enabled to give feedback to risk assessors when an assessment is out of date. If a Person has a condition which is likely to deteriorate, then reassessment should be frequent - perhaps a weekly review. Managers should also check with their care

Personal Handling Profile

This form should be used in conjunction with the risk factor check list.

Name	
Assessor	
Signature	
Date Assessed	
Proposed Review Date *(every 6 months unless condition alters)*	

Summary of Person's physical condition and handling constraints including any relevant medical diagnosis

Approximate weight, height and build of Person

Any other considerations (e.g. personal/family preferences & opinions)

Identify any problems with communication, comprehension or behaviour

Sign and date the change alert column to indicate a change has occurred. Refer to update sheet

Tasks No. & description	Details of method to be used including any equipment & techniques	Change Alert
		Cont. overleaf

Safer Handling of People in the Community

Tasks No. & description	Details of method to be used including any equipment & techniques	Change Alert

Is there any equipment required to safely perform any of the tasks? Give details

Where will the equipment be obtained?	
Date requested and by whom	

Please check that you have given details of action required if no equipment available *

Is there any follow-up action required (e.g. staff training, OT referral)? Give details

Please organise relevant follow up action now! *

Describe any remaining problems/risk factors using the 'LITE' approach

Update Sheet

Add any changes to previous methods

Date	Task No.	Details of updated method to be used	Signature

staff whether a Person's situation has changed and should be quick to respond to a request for a reassessment.

Generic risk assessment

A useful way to help identify key areas of concern and implement safer systems of work is to carry out a generic assessment. This involves assessing tasks which are similar and common to the workforce as a whole. By assessing these tasks, general procedures using safer systems of work can be implemented.

A home care team will need to move People in bed on a regular basis. A generic assessment will broadly consider the problems that can be encountered with this task and how to minimise risk in many instances. The manager can then ensure that carers have access to equipment in advance of a situation, have procedures and guidelines to follow according to the findings of the Personal Handling Profile (PHP) and clearly set standards for certain manoeuvres etc.

When using this 'generic assessment' however, it is important to check that the Person concerned really does fit into the general procedure, or else make appropriate amendments. It may be necessary to outline short- and long-term action if changes cannot be implemented immediately.

Use of agency staff

A care manager's knowledge of the abilities and limitations of care staff under his or her management will never be complete. It is for this reason that, even if they are responsible for doing the risk assessment, a senior carer or care worker will still have to review the entire assessment to ensure the staff have the knowledge, skills and ability to do the job. With agency staff, the care manager knows even less and has far less control over the standard of care that will be provided. Whether they are in statutory ot independent organisations, care managers, including those involved with hospital discharge, must liaise and communicate regularly to ensure that every carer meets the same standards and follows similar procedures. It may be useful to have training in moving and handling and risk assessment which employees in statutory authorities and agency staff attend. This also helps each group understand their respective strengths and weaknesses, and helps pave the way for more consistency of care for the Person who is, after all, often paying for this service. Managers, however, must bear in mind that they are responsible for ensuring all staff, including agency staff, have had appropriate training. They are not responsible for providing training for agency staff; that is the agency's responsibility.

Summary

Prior to providing care, the risk assessor needs to ensure that risks are minimised to the lowest level reasonably practicable and that there is a safe system of work in place for all carers. The system of work must be monitored, reviewed and updated as necessary. All changes must be documented. The key points below may help managers with their assessments.

Be In Control

We cannot remove all the hazards from our workplace but we need to minimise the risk they pose to the lowest level possible. We need to aim to be in control of the hazards that are in our workplace rather than be forced to furiously bail out after an accident happens.

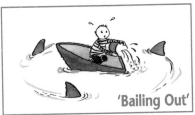 'Bailing Out'

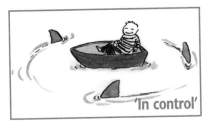 'In control'

(Reproduced with kind permission of the HSE)

KEY POINTS

1   As a manager you have a duty to make sure a general risk assessment and a Personal Handling Profile has been undertaken for every Person needing assistance to move. This will include:

♦ identifying hazards (potential dangers)

♦ identifying who is at risk

♦ evaluating the risks - is enough being done to control the hazards?

2   You need to act on the findings of your assessment to reduce the risks to all those involved:

♦ document all findings

♦ implement prevention and control measures; seek external advice from therapists, carers and Moving and Handling or Back Care Advisers

♦ use a generic risk assessment to provide a standard for common tasks.

3   Having undertaken the risk assessments, you need to ensure that all staff follow them:

♦ inform all staff of the procedures and check they can all follow the system of work in place.

4   The assessments need to be reviewed regularly as the Person's condition changes (e.g. every six months):

♦ monitor and review; use the carers to provide feedback.

REMEMBER - BE PROACTIVE, NOT REACTIVE.

REFERENCES

HSE, (1998). *Guidance on Manual Handling Operations Regulations. HMSO, London.*

National Back Pain Association, (1997). *The Guide to the Handling of Patients, Fourth Edition. National Back Pain Association in collaboration with the Royal College of Nursing, London.*

RCN, (1995). *Patient Handling Standards - Checklist of risk factors. Royal College of Nursing, London.*

RCN, (1996). *Manual Handling Assessments in Hospital and the Community - an RCN guide. Royal College of Nursing, London.*

FURTHER READING

Department of Health (Social Services Inspectorate),(1993). *No Longer Afraid - The safeguard of older people in domestic settings. HMSO, London.*

Department of Health (Social Services Inspectorate),(1995). *Caring for people at home. HMSO, London.*

HSE, (1999). *Five steps to Risk Assessment. HMSO, London.*

4 Training - Why is it important?

Clive Tracey

Introduction

Training in moving and handling is a vital aspect of implementing safe systems of work for staff. However, managers cannot rely on manual handling training alone to fulfil their statutory obligations. Training should be used in conjunction with safer work practices, and the level and content of training will depend upon the risk reduction measures adopted.

THE EMPLOYER'S DUTY

Employers have a general duty under Section 2.2 of the Health & Safety at Work Act, 1974 (HSWA, 1974) to provide suitable and sufficient information, instruction, training and supervision to safeguard the health, safety and welfare of their staff while at work (See Chapter 1: Legislation and Responsibilities). The scope of this training is not clear, but there is a requirement for training to be provided **before** staff are exposed to a hazard, or if the level of risk changes. Staff, therefore, require training on induction, if new equipment or work practices are introduced, and on a regular basis.

Frequency and duration of training

The Health and Safety Commission's Services Advisory Committee [HSAC] recommends that training is provided on an annual basis if the skills are to be retained or kept up to date. It advises that 'professional trainers' expect at least 2 days training for inexperienced staff but this may increase to 3 - 5 days (HSC,1992). The correct amount of training time is variable and will depend on: the issues to be covered (see Content of Training below page 49); the number of staff to be trained, their experience and skills. Training time has been successfully split or reduced where alternative sources of advice, training or support are available, for example with staff who have a key worker able to reinforce safer practices. If staff have no support in the workplace, they need to acquire all their skills through the formal training sessions. Key workers will need more intensive training. It is unlikely they will develop the necessary assessment skills, problem-solving ability, and knowledge of a range of techniques and equipment in courses of less than 4 days duration.

Ultimately, the question to consider before you decide how much time should be allocated is:

WHAT IS THE TRAINING TRYING TO ACHIEVE?

For example:

♦ If your staff are exposed to complex handling situations, and are expected to deal with them, the time you give for training needs to be longer to allow these skills to be developed.

♦ Training may be limited if it is to complement other systems or address specific issues (e.g. training in the use of a new hoist).

Training should not be a substitute for implementing other risk reduction measures. So you can't give longer training instead of providing proper equipment.

OTHER FACTORS

Organisational culture

An important influencing factor is the culture of the organisation including the attitudes of staff. For example, if staff are opposed to changing the way they have always moved people, then you need to spend time exploring these attitudes before you start training on specific techniques.

Handling policies

Problems that care staff might face when translating policy into practice should be addressed in training. If, as has been outlined in Chapter 1(see pages 12-14), the local policy is written clearly and sensibly, problems and conflicts are far less likely to occur. With the introduction of the Manual Handling Operations Regulations 1992 [MHOR, 1992] and their endorsement by the Royal College of Nursing through their 'Safer Handling Policy' (RCN, 1996), training is now seen as a way to limit or root out unsafe practices. The training concentrates on a limited set of techniques that do not involve taking all or most of a person's weight. Training sessions tend to be run over one or more days, mixing theory and practice. The benefit of this is that staff gain an understanding of the principles of safer handling, and are able to question, rather than merely learning new skills. Progressive organisations that have implemented alternative programmes for risk reduction (e.g. electrically operated beds, hoisting equipment and changes in work patterns), have, in some cases, successfully reduced training to half a day. However, this is not an adequate training time if the training is provided in isolation from other methods of education and support, such as the key worker system.

Awareness raising

Current thinking amongst some Back Care Advisers is that general awareness of safer practices plus work-based problem-solving is an alternative to conventional training. It avoids lengthy, inadequate training on techniques that may not be the solution to the risks to which staff are exposed.

Content of training programmes

1 ERGONOMIC PRINCIPLES AND CONCEPTS

It is essential that you make staff aware of all the factors that may increase the risk of injury when moving an object or Person. The ergonomic approach advocated by the MHOR, (HSE, 1992) is highlighted under the heading LITE (see Chapter 3: Assessing Risks).

LOAD: The Person or object that has to be moved.

INDIVIDUAL: Who is providing the care.

TASK: What has to be done, how and when.

ENVIRONMENT: Where the Person is being cared for.

2 SPINAL ANATOMY AND CAUSES OF INJURY

Your staff will not fully appreciate those principles if they do not understand the function, structure and movement of the spine (see Chapter 2: Principles of Safer Handling). The more that staff are aware of the causes of back injuries in their area of work, the more they are able to influence the adoption of measures to reduce risk (e.g. the purchase of hi/lo baths to prevent awkward and static postures while assisting someone in the bath).

3 BACK FACTS

Allied to this, staff may take more notice when they see the startling statistics for back injuries, lost time at work and the associated costs. It is beneficial if these figures can be related to or compared with their own sphere of work.

4 LEGAL ISSUES

Everyone needs to be aware of their legal responsibilities and of the framework of law which surrounds manual handling. Staff need to take responsibility for their own actions and for the environment in which they are working. They need to be in control.

5 PRINCIPLES OF SAFER HANDLING

The golden rules of **avoid, assess** and **reduce** must be followed in any plan of action. A summary list may help your staff remember the key points.

1 Avoid manual lifting where possible.

2 Assess what needs to be done.

3 Assess the situation, the Person or object to be moved.

4 Use equipment whenever possible to reduce the risk of injury.

5 Know your limitations and get help if necessary.

6 Communicate with all team members and the Person who is being moved.

7 Prepare the area.

8 Adopt a correct position following principles of good body mechanics (see Chapter 2: Principles of Safer Handling).

9 Always keep the load close to the body.

10 Control the move - keep it smooth and balanced.

6 AIDS AND EQUIPMENT

Most risk reduction programmes will involve the introduction of aids (see Chapter 6: Equipment). You must support their introduction with training in their use and selection as well as their suitability, availability and maintenance. You need to reinforce the benefits of using equipment, how to operate it, and refresh this regularly, at least on a yearly basis.

7 TECHNIQUES

It is no good just saying "Don't do it this way!". You need to give staff alternatives. Techniques, including the use of equipment, must follow the basic biomechanical principles as follows:

KEEP THE

♦ load close to the body

♦ spine with natural curves present

♦ knees bent.

Knees should be bent especially if starting or finishing at a low level. Back care advisers have expressed concern that this may just move the injury site from the back to other parts of the body (i.e. knees and shoulders). However, the structure and design of these joints mean that they are better able to tolerate stress. Full squatting is not recommended as taking one's weight on the balls of the feet in this way is unstable. Having your knee fully bent also makes it much more difficult for the thigh muscles to raise the body weight.

The techniques demonstrated should complement the use of a range of handling aids in various situations. Staff should be allowed to practise new skills under supervision. It is recommended that there is one trainer to every six students. This allows time for practice with adequate supervision. However, most training sessions only allow one pair of staff to practise at any one time under the direct supervision of a trainer. In this situation the ratio is unimportant, but an increase in the class size will require more time for students to practise and demonstrate their ability to correctly perform the technique.

The most important aspect of teaching a skill is that you need to make sure the staff member is able to perform the skill before leaving the class and that records have been completed (see below, page 54). Finally, no student should feel they must join in a practical skill or practice demonstrations if they do not feel confident, or if they feel that a physical problem of their own may be made worse. In this situation, you may need to refer the staff member back to their line manager or the Occupational Health Department.

8 KEEP IT RELEVANT

Whatever training is given, the knowledge level and content must be suitable and realistic for the staff group being trained. It is all too easy to talk about ideals that do not work or cannot be applied in the real situations which trainees will face in practice.

9 THE TRAINERS

There is presently an Inter-Professional Curriculum to train trainers approved by the main professional bodies, the Ergonomic Society and National Back Exchange (NBE, 1995). This syllabus will equip trainers, and those responsible for implementing an organisation's strategy for 'manual handling', with the appropriate skills. Local programmes should follow this syllabus.

Delivering Training

Many employers and managers cite time pressures and the inability to release staff as a hindrance to the provision of training. This is not an acceptable excuse. There are a several ways you can organise training.

1 DIRECT TRAINING

This involves a designated trainer with the appropriate experience and knowledge to deliver all the training. It ensures that the quality and content of the training is consistent and that all staff receive the same information. It also eliminates the need to release a member of staff from the work area to act as trainer. It does, however, create reliance on one person and if that person leaves, it may be costly to employ another trainer or pay freelance fees.

2 CASCADE TRAINER SYSTEM

In certain situations, cascade training can be a useful way of getting information to all staff quickly. However, it is often misunderstood. Pure cascading is where staff are trained, who in turn train others and so on down the line. This system must be avoided for manual handling training, as the skills are diluted, and unsafe practices are likely to result. However, one level of cascade may be appropriate for some organisations which wish to keep knowledge and skills in-house. The trainer is generally part of the workforce and, therefore, needs to attend a course to gain the relevant skills. The problem here is that there are currently no national standards, although the Inter-Professional Curriculum (NBE, 1995) aims to address this omission. There may be cost benefits: the cost is for each nominated trainer's course fees only, plus the cost of releasing them from their normal work.

3 DIRECT/KEY WORKER SYSTEM

Experience has shown this to be an effective combination. Training is delivered by a designated trainer and then reinforced and supported in the workplace by key workers. Key workers are also available to enforce good practice and help solve problems at a more local level. Larger organisations use two trainers per session, allowing a greater number of staff to be trained (12 staff and a 6:1 ratio). This has the additional benefit that techniques requiring two carers can be safely taught (with only one trainer, a student is used and this may put both student and trainer at risk). The skills and confidence of the key workers may be developed, while ensuring the quality of the training is maintained. This is a potentially costly system but the benefits of having support within the workplace and securing high quality training are well worth the expense. Larger organisations are also able to train all their staff within a realistic time frame. The system is further improved with the support of central booking and record keeping.

Supervision and demonstrations within the workplace are highly effective as staff immediately see the relevance to their work. However, on the job training should not be the sole method of training, and it must never put People at risk from inappropriately skilled trainers practising with them. Teaching, using People in real situations without involving them properly in the process, should not be accepted as good practice. A further problem is that the training is often limited to one specific issue and hence record-keeping becomes complex. It may also be costly as it is normally delivered on a one-to-one basis. The system is useful within People's homes when equipment is delivered to ensure the staff and the Person are familiar with its use.

Organisational Issues

A strategy for 'manual handling' should be detailed within the organisation's policy and approved at a senior level. No system will achieve the required results unless there is a firm commitment to implementing safer systems. Key issues that often arise are discussed below.

1 RELEASING STAFF

This is the most common problem for any training programme. The timing has to suit the working practices - some residential homes or departments may be able to close for specific periods while others increase staff numbers or release staff during a handover period. It is often easier if training can be contained in one day allowing sufficient cover to be organised rather than trying to cope with less staff on a busy shift.

A day incorporating the mandatory training of Health & Safety, Fire, Manual Handling and Resuscitation has been highly successful in increasing staff numbers attending at King's Healthcare NHS Trust, London. Previously the training was offered independently and staff found it difficult to attend for 1 - 3 hours during a shift. Cost savings have been seen in the form of less training time needed and there has also been improved management information from accurate records.

However, training has to be geared to the needs of staff. This means that it may not always be possible to provide training between 9.00am and 5.00pm. Many shift workers or part-time workers are not available during a standard working day, but their need for training must not be overlooked.

Another way is for a number of nursing homes to group together, sharing the cost of the training day, each releasing one or two staff members. This limits the disruption to each home and ensures the training is cost-effective provided the maximum numbers attend each session.

2 BOOKING

Smaller organisations may have an easier task in planning programmes and ensuring that all staff attend. Employers with a large number of staff or departments may find it difficult. A simple central booking system can ease the burden. You need to ensure that the system provides all the participants with any pre-course information in time, and that they have given adequate notice if the session needs to be changed in any way (e.g. venue) or cancelled for any reason. A database allows reference for statistics and reporting. In addition, it can identify when staff require training, thus easing the burden on managers.

3 RECORDS

Any training given to staff must be recorded and the records kept for future reference. Records are important: to show compliance with statutory requirements, to highlight content covered, and for statistical analysis. They are a check, and are used in legal cases either by the employer, to show that adequate training was given, or by the staff member, to demonstrate that the training did not meet their needs and address the specific issue against which they are claiming. Incomplete records are not useful. There are a number of different records:

♦ Register: This is a record of people attending. It does not record individual performance or techniques practised. The register should include individual records and trainer notes (see below).

♦ Individual records: This is completed by each staff member and is a record of what was demonstrated to them and what they practised.

♦ Trainer notes: The notes used for each session should be kept, or a record made if a standard package has been used. If changes are made to the notes then the old notes should be kept. It is useful to keep a record of what was actually covered in each session and a note if staff members were unable to perform tasks, arrived late or other issues arose which would not be covered by the other records.

Training Centre

The person responsible for organising and providing training needs to do the following tasks.

1. Set the appropriate time for training. This will depend on the criteria outlined above, the content of the training, the number of students and issues to be addressed.

2. Ensure that resources that are needed such as equipment, visual aids and handouts are organised.

3. Ensure all staff receive training, and that training is repeated and refreshed on an annual basis.

4. Establish and maintain a record system, which may be aided by a database. Provide regular reports for managers to enable them to monitor the progress of their staff.

5. Develop and provide training courses comprising:

   ♦ awareness raising

   ♦ legal issues

   ♦ biomechanics

   ♦ ergonomics

   ♦ assessments of People

   ♦ principles of safer moving and handling

   ♦ techniques for moving inanimate objects

   ♦ techniques for moving People.

The benefits of training

As has been demonstrated throughout this chapter, training complements any other system that reduces the risk of injury, such as the provision of hoisting equipment or electrically-operated beds. Training will ensure that staff are safer when using equipment and that risk reduction is achieved. Training is a complex area. On its own, training has little effect in reducing the risk of injury. The use of training to raise staff awareness, combined with the introduction of equipment or changes in work practices should be encouraged. Training should give staff the ability to say 'NO'. Although it is a legal requirement with recommended content, the way it is achieved in each organisation will be different, according to local resources and the level of commitment to safer practices. Training is highly effective if planned correctly and supported; if not, it can be a costly waste of effort.

REFERENCES

Chartered Society of Physiotherapy (CSP), (1996). When to delegate tasks. Information Paper No. PA6. CSP, London.

HSC, (1992). Management of Health and Safety at Work: Approved Code of Practice. HMSO, London.

HSC, (1998). Guidance on the Manual Handling of Loads in the Health Services. HMSO, London.

HSE, (1998). Guidance on Manual Handling Operations Regulations. HMSO, London.

National Back Pain Association, (1998). The Guide to the Handling of Patients, Fourth Edition. National Back Pain Association in collaboration with the Royal College of Nursing, London.

National Back Exchange, (1995). Inter-Professional Curriculum. In association with the Chartered Society of Physiotherapists, the College of Occupational Therapists, the Ergonomic Society and the Royal College of Nursing. Scutari Projects, Harrow, Middlesex.

Royal College of Nursing, (1996). Code of Practice for Patient Handling. RCN, London.

Royal College of Nursing, (1996). Introducing a Safer Patient Handling Policy. RCN, London.

UK Government, (1974). Health and Safety at Work etc. Act. HMSO, London.

5 The Person and the environment

Patricia P Wright, Sally Cassar and Liz Aitchison

Introduction

Much of the language surrounding 'moving and handling' is very impersonal, and anyone involved in providing care and support to another Person needs to keep in mind who that Person is. In this chapter, we take a brief look at some of the wider aspects of caring for People in the community, issues of the Person and the environment. Caring for others creates a relationship between people based on a level of dependence that is not mutually balanced. Essentially, one Person needs something that the other person provides. Caring for others can also create a relationship that is intensely personal and sometimes very intimate. Further, it can require the formation of several interconnected relationships, as the carer works alongside informal carers, relatives or friends. All sorts of People may need help: People of all ages, races and religions; People with a range of disabilities, both temporary and permanent; People who live within strong family and social networks and People who are alone. A fundamental part of the carer's task is to *empower* each Person, whatever their particular circumstances, to regain as much control of their own life as possible. This will also contribute to the goal of safer working.

The chapter is divided into four sections. The first outlines core values which should inform the work of a carer in the community. In the second section we look at how these core values can be put into practice, offering some general guidelines to help carers to approach the People with whom they work. We also offer some examples of issues that may arise working with People with acute degenerative or chronic conditions. We cover briefly social and cultural issues to highlight the need to be sensitive to the Person's broader situation and history. Thirdly, we take a practical look at some of the points to bear in mind when changes have to be made in a Person's home. Finally, we offer some tips to help carers to remain fit for the challenges of their work.

Core values

The Department of Health has described a set of core values for community care:

♦ that People should be treated as individuals

♦ that each Person should have equal access to service provision regardless of race, gender or disability

♦ that a Person should be allowed to remain independent and have a right to take risks

♦ that a Person's privacy should be respected

♦ that respect should be given for a Person's need for dignity and individuality

♦ that a Person should be able to have an individual choice of services

♦ that People should be allowed to achieve their own goals.

(Care Management: Summary of Practice Guidelines, 1992 (Para 81))

Putting core values into practice

Communication, awareness and sensitivity are the basic building blocks which must inform your attitude if you are to offer successful and safe care.

COMMUNICATION

The importance of good communication at every stage cannot be emphasised enough. From the initial point of assessing needs to the carrying out of each element of care day by day, communication is vital. First and foremost, you must know what the Person's wishes are, and develop the care plan in partnership with the Person for whom it is intended, and anyone else who is significantly involved in the overall task of providing care. You must fully explain it so that the Person understands what is planned and has confidence in it. You need to ensure a similar level of mutual agreement from the family so that safe practice can be carried out at all times. Some People may be reluctant to accept help and this reluctance may intensify if it is necessary to change the home environment in order to ensure safer practice (see below, page 69). Good communication is vital as part of a carer's approach to reducing risk. By explaining clearly what needs to be done, how and why, you can help to minimise the unexpected - communication prepares both parties.

It must be remembered that communication is a two-way process. You must always offer People the opportunity to express how they would like to be cared for. Sometimes there are extra challenges, for instance when you are caring for People with sensory loss (deafness or failing sight) or some level of learning disability. You should discuss the extent of the disability and methods used to deal with it at the time of assessment. A Person with a hearing impairment, for example, may not use their hearing aid due to pain or discomfort in the ear, or they may use signing or lip reading to communicate. If they use lip reading, it will be pointless to try to tell them what to do when you are at their side. It is important to develop a workable communication system and explain what will happen in advance. A tap on the Person's forearm to signal when certain things need to happen can be effective. A very important tool is pen and paper - a brief written explanation or a diagram of what will be happening can help. In the case of a Person with a sight problem, they need to be aware of where items of equipment have been placed and you should ask their help in suggesting a safe location. As well as letting the Person know where the equipment is, you should also encourage them to feel all the component parts so that they can imagine the item.

Following a stroke, a Person may lose the ability to speak but this does not mean they are unable to understand what is going on around them. You need to have a great deal of patience in explaining what has happened and what is planned. To help prevent the frustration felt by a Person who has suffered a stroke, you can use a communication system such as charts of words and pictures. In many situations, you may also have to explain things *several times*, repeating previous explanations and taking care to be very patient.

AWARENESS AND SENSITIVITY

As a carer, you need to be aware that every Person to whom you offer support is different. Each Person needs to be considered holistically, that is in the context of their *whole life*, not just their recent experience of illness or disability. There is much written to help you understand the implications of specific physical or psychological conditions. But you should also consider the Person's history, their cultural background, their religious beliefs, and social expectations. However, guard against making general assumptions based on your own personal views, for example, of how a particular condition will affect a particular Person. The Person should be the primary source of information about their special needs at the time of the assessment. By making an accurate assessment of how they usually carry out the activities of daily living you can help to determine what assistance they need. A sensitive approach will enable suitable adjustments to be built into the individual care plan.

Being sensitive to People's anxiety

It is very important you are aware that, each Person who needs care, whatever their illness or disability, is likely to feel some degree of anxiety or fear as a result of their changed situation. Such fears may be temporary because the condition is short-lived or because they are able to adjust to their new circumstances. However, anxiety may also be ongoing or recurring; it may even be a part of the illness itself. Dealing with People who are anxious or fearful is an integral part of your role and requires a high level of patience and sensitivity. For many People, calm, clear and reassuring communication will allay most of their fears. It is also important that you have a positive approach, for example when suggesting changes in the home or the use of equipment. You need to explain, for example, how the introduction of a hoist can enable a Person to be helped to and from bed in a comfortable and dignified manner. You must also make the Person aware of the choices they may have, for instance by showing them the different types of hoists which are available, so that they can feel involved in choosing the one most appropriate for their situation. If the Person is able to visit a Disabled Living Centre, all types of equipment can be explained and demonstrated to them. However, remember that the hoist of choice should also meet the needs of the carer and of key members of the family, or friends who may be playing a major role in caring for the Person.

Sometimes, a fear or lack of understanding of what is happening to them can lead to aggression in People whose lives have been disrupted by illness or trauma. Patience in explaining fully how you plan to care for them should alleviate their anxiety and reduce this risk. At all times, your approach should be appropriate to the Person's specific needs and circumstances. It may help if you engage other family members or close friends in this process; they may retain the trust and confidence of the Person and, by working together to provide reassurance, the aggressive feelings may be dissipated. If you are unable to find a way of dealing with challenging or aggressive behaviour, you might discuss specific issues with the Person's primary worker. This may be a Community Psychiatric Nurse or Psychiatric Social Worker. The care plan should give specific examples of what may cause the Person to become aggressive, thus enabling the carer to avoid situations which may provoke aggression; for example, they may dislike their 'personal space' being invaded, or have a fear or dislike of certain topics being discussed.

Different needs - different challenges

Many People may need extra care and support at some stage in their lives because of illness or temporary disability, or because their partner or primary carer has become ill themselves. A healthy Person who suffers an episode which prevents them from carrying out the activities of daily living may need help in the short term. Equally, such a Person may be left with a significant level of chronic disability and need support in the longer term. Here we will consider some of the different demands and challenges of acute, degenerative and chronic conditions.

ACUTE CONDITIONS

An acute condition is one where symptoms occur suddenly and are often severe but of a short duration, as in the case of acute bronchitis or acute pain. Acute illnesses may have many causes, such as infection or following surgery, and can be physical or mental illnesses. The Person may feel weak and perhaps listless, preferring to remain in bed. While rest and recuperation are very important, they must be combined with an active mobilisation programme as quickly as possible to prevent complications occurring or the condition becoming chronic. Following an operation, People are now expected to get out of bed within a few hours, to prevent complications such as thrombosis. Early discharge from hospital means that many People need help in their own homes. For a Person who is usually healthy, only limited help for certain activities may be needed, for example, bathing. However, where a Person has a pre-existing condition, such as arthritis or a heart condition, more help may be required. The Person may need help with bathing, dressing or using the toilet. If the Person is unable to walk unaided, it may help them to have a commode beside their bed and perhaps use a walking frame to enable them to move without undue stress to the carer. People are sometimes reluctant to use such aids but you should encourage them to do so to help them maintain their independence. Extra encouragement can be given by informal carers or members of the family. Your objective should be to return the Person to independent living as soon as possible.

In the past, many People have become dependent upon services because time was not spent in encouraging them to do as much as possible for themselves in the initial stages of the illness. Pain upon moving, which is often a symptom of an acute condition, can make a Person reluctant to move. You should look for ways of reducing such pain; perhaps an analgesic can be prescribed and given in time to relieve pain when carrying out certain procedures. This will reduce the risk of injuries to both the Person and the carer.

Sudden illness such as a **stroke** may be classified as an acute condition, especially if there is the prospect of significant improvement in functional ability over time. People who have suffered a stroke must be allowed to try to do as much as they can for themselves, even though it may take longer. It is very easy to make a Person dependent by, for example, buttoning shirts or cardigans, rather than showing them how to do this for themselves. Setting small simple steps or goals will encourage progress. If the task you set is too hard and the Person is unable to achieve it, they may become very discouraged or depressed, and this may delay improvement in their condition. Depression is often a complicating factor when a Person with a stroke cannot understand what has happened or what their future will be. Depression is, in any case, a normal reaction to a significant loss. The loss of functional ability, whether temporary or permanent, is something that the Person and their relatives need to grieve over. Unless it is worked through adequately and with the necessary support, depression can result.

Schizophrenia is a mental illness which affects all aspects of the Person's life, including the way they think, how they feel and the way they behave. One of the greatest difficulties is that the Person may be unaware that something is wrong. They find it difficult to decide what is real and what is not. It is often described as like having a dream while being awake. People with schizophrenia are not usually violent or dangerous; more often they are timid and frightened. When needs are assessed, it is important that you are aware that they are probably unable, rather than unwilling to co-operate with any plans for their care. Stress and emotional pressure can exacerbate symptoms during the course of the illness and, therefore, care should be taken to talk through quietly and gently what is required to help them. Until treatment becomes fully effective, you may have problems persuading the Person to co-operate in meeting their physical care needs. This requires much patience on your part and repeated explanations of what is happening, until the symptoms of the illness improve. This highlights the need for awareness of the progress of an illness to ensure that you are able to care fully and safely for the Person.

DEGENERATIVE CONDITIONS

The key feature of these conditions is that they are progressive. However, their progress may not be steady and there may be periods when the Person is able to move themselves with little or no help, interspersed with periods of greater dependence. Many conditions develop gradually, as with arthritis and degenerative changes in the spine. In degenerative conditions, the normal structure and functioning of cells and tissues is damaged or lost. This may be due to death or decay of cells or nerves.

Examples

Motor Neurone Disease is an example where there is a gradual effect on the abilities of the Person to care for themselves. Initial weakness or loss of movement in limbs can reduce mobility; later this will progress to complete loss of use of the affected muscles. The care plan needs to allow for these gradual changes and you need to reassure the Person by explaining what kinds of help will be available to them. In the initial stages of a degenerative condition, the Person may require only minimal help but as the condition progresses, increasing input from outside carers will be required.

Multiple sclerosis is a degenerative condition that can often present difficulties in assessment of needs, as the progress of the illness can be very erratic. Initial assessments should take into account that remission periods often occur and that it is important to allow People to care for themselves when they are able to do so. However, a plan should be in place to enable a Person to call upon services when they need them. This can be difficult when service provision has to be prioritised. It may be that People refuse services which do not meet their immediate needs, perhaps because they find it difficult to face up to or accept their condition, or have an unrealistic expectation that the family will carry the burden of care. It is important that you work with the family to ensure that their needs are understood. If help is not offered as quickly as possible, there may be an acute breakdown within the family.

Alzheimer's disease is usually associated with older People, although it is not unknown in younger adults. It is a progressive mental illness, starting with loss of short-term memory and forgetfulness, and progresses to the Person being unable to take responsibility for everyday self-care needs. This may take place over a matter of months or years, and there may be periods when the Person can think clearly and is able to care for themselves. When assessing needs relating to moving and handling, it is important that you know at what stage of the illness the Person may be. People with advanced Alzheimer's disease may have problems with walking as well as caring for themselves generally. A Person who is confused may lack understanding of their safety needs. If this is the case, you will need to be patient when explaining how the type of equipment you are proposing will be used; again, the help of informal carers in reinforcing this message is vital. There may be serious issues about individual safety to be considered, although it should be remembered that independence must be maintained as much as possible.

Many diseases, which occur as a result of the **ageing process**, may occur very gradually and are not always apparent to the Person or their families. On the other hand, depression and minor physical illnesses, such as urinary infections, can cause symptoms which are mistaken for, or assumed to be degenerative conditions. It is important that a continuous review is made so that appropriate care can be introduced before accidents happen. People who have degenerative illness require constant review of their condition and needs. A major factor here is that the Person may experience emotional problems and deny that anything is the matter and this may affect how you are able to care for them. They may become difficult, demanding and depressed when they are trying to deal with the issues surrounding the progress of the illness.

Care of **terminally ill** People at home, or in a residential care home, may be interspersed with hospice care. You must ensure that adequate help and support is provided at all stages to enable People to have the confidence to remain in a familiar environment as long as possible. There may be occasions when, as the Person's condition deteriorates, additional equipment will have to be proposed. For anyone who has slept in the same bed as their partner for many years, it may be very distressing if a profiling/hospital type bed needs to be brought into the home. Explaining the advantages to both the Person and their partner in terms of comfort and safety of care may help. Objections may, for example, be overcome by suggesting that the single bed be placed beside the lowered profiling bed so that a degree of intimacy and comfort can be retained. The profiling bed can then be raised for carrying out care. The Person and their family should be made aware that this is necessary for the safety of both the Person and the carer.

People who are terminally ill may be very tired or in pain, therefore visits by care staff should be planned to make the most of the time when pain relief is given to ensure their comfort when they are being moved. It is often assumed that frail and debilitated People will not be difficult to move. In fact, the opposite is usually the case since the Person may be unable to help themselves very much. This creates additional stress on the carer's back. As the illness progresses, the Person may become unable to stand alone, therefore you must continually assess the care routine to reduce the risk of accidents.

CHRONIC CONDITIONS

A chronic condition is an illness of long duration usually of gradual onset and often difficult to treat, for example, chronic pain. It may or may not be severe. Due to the long period of time over which a condition becomes chronic, it can cause many problems which have implications for moving and handling.

Examples

A condition such as **rheumatoid arthritis**, which has an effect on the joints of the body, is a good example. Pain is a major feature of the disease. This can create a problem for the carer when helping to move the Person as they may be reluctant to be moved due to the extent of the pain. It is important that you encourage the Person to explain what causes them particular distress and try to suggest ways of helping them move which will minimise their pain.

Chronic pain can be one of the most tricky conditions you may encounter. Following an illness or injury the main cause of the pain may have disappeared, for example in the case of someone who has had a limb amputated. While the affected part of the body has been removed, the brain may continue to receive messages that the previous cause of the pain is still there. This can be very distressing and confusing for the Person and they may have difficulties in coming to terms with the loss of the limb when they continue to feel the pain. In some situations, for example with People who suffer from chronic back pain, the original cause of the pain may have been removed. Pain is there to indicate that there is a problem. The nature of pain changes with time and, following the initial healing of soft tissue, pain can continue, becoming severe and incapacitating, while not always having an obvious physical explanation. This may cause increasing distress and depression. One of the factors of pain is that the Person may be reluctant to move the affected part of the body. This in turn results in weakness or, if left for too long, atrophy* of muscles, and can have a devastating effect on mobility.

A chronic condition which affects the heart and lungs may give rise to difficulties with breathing and will limit the Person's ability to fulfil daily living activities. **Emphysema** or a **chronic heart condition** for example, can affect the ability to breathe properly; therefore simple activities such as getting to the bathroom or even getting up from a chair will present a major problem. In addition to the anxieties about the disease itself, the issues about being dependent upon someone else for care can be very distressing for the Person and for the people close to them. You should be aware of how their condition affects the Person not only

---

* Atrophy: see Glossary

physically but also emotionally and mentally. There may be a support group in your area, details of which will be available from your Area Health Authority. It is important to remember that family members and their informal carers may also need external support. Carers' or Relatives' groups may also exist locally and details of these can usually be found in libraries.

People with extensive chronic disabilities will still require an approach that offers opportunities for choice. An individual assessment will identify their specific needs. A Person with **dementia,** for example, may be reluctant, through disorientation, or a lack of insight or understanding, to co-operate with plans for bathing and/or the use of the toilet. Rather than bathing a Person in a bed or chair, it might be better to suggest that you wash them while they sit on a toilet or a commode with a bidet-type seat, to reduce the amount of moving. You might find that kneeling on a suitable comfortable and protected surface, with items required immediately to hand, reduces the stress on your back. Chronic conditions may often require permanent use of equipment in the home. Older People may be reluctant to accept help, especially if the use of handling equipment is proposed. Although you would hope to respect their wishes, you should make it clear they refuse equipment which is necessary for their and your safety, the level of help provided may be restricted.

An important consideration for you to bear in mind is that while a Person has an illness for which they require your help, they remain the individual that they were before the illness. They remain a person who is important to their family, friends and colleagues. They have fears, emotions and value to the community.

BEING SENSITIVE TO PEOPLE'S CULTURE

People needing care come from a wide variety of social, ethnic and cultural backgrounds. You should try to find out as much as possible about the specific requirements which People may have as a result before the assessment takes place. At the same time, you must avoid making generalisations based on background research or previous experience. These can be misleading. For example, some People may expect intimate care to be undertaken by close family or professionals, while other help could come from other carers. However, such expectations vary within and across cultural groupings (Sinclair et al, 1998). The Person should be consulted closely at the time of the assessment. So, too, should the family and other key people. Although there are many People who are isolated, without family or friends, the majority live within some kind of network. It is important to understand the expectations of those key people and they can provide important details to help ensure that People are supported sensitively. Your 'normal' routine for visiting People in their own homes may need to be reviewed, for example to respect different religious festivals and holidays, or to allow for prayer or meditation, which may take place at regular intervals during the day. Again, if you take a sensitive approach you will be able to incorporate suitable adjustments into the care plan. Some ethnic communities have certain practices that must be followed and others that are optional or should be avoided. It may also be helpful to consult alternative sources of information, such as local community groups. It is difficult to provide a comprehensive list of national or local organisations, however, this information should be available from local information sources such as the Citizens Advice Bureau or Community Relations Council.

Religious beliefs

In some cultures and religious groups, particular emphasis is placed upon prayer. For example, in the Hindu faith prayer takes place after bathing in the morning and people of working age will rise early for this purpose. An older Person may rise later and the family may not allow visits to interrupt their prayers. Traditionally in the Jewish community, men pray three times per day for up to 30 minutes or longer on the Sabbath (Friday evening and Saturday morning), as well as 5 to 10 minutes during the afternoon and evening. The very religious will not take a meal before prayer. Prayers should not be interrupted unless medically necessary. You should therefore pay particular attention to times and places of prayer or meditation as well as any special festivals in order to avoid offence. Communicating why you may need to visit at these times is essential.

Attitude to family

In many cultures, great emphasis is placed on family life, and carers need to be able to create partnerships with family members and work within the network of close extended families. The professional carer is joining with, and adding to the caring being done by others. Carers need to remember that these people undertake the bulk of care. In some religions, such as Islam, there is a strong commitment to care for older People whether they are related or not; older People are not encouraged to live alone, and the idea of the extended family is a fundamental one that Muslims will try to maintain. This must influence your approach if there is a need to persuade People to accept care from outside when they most need it. While there is an expectation within a family that they will care for each other, it must not be assumed that families can meet all of their own needs. Some People refuse care from outside carers as they say that their partners, families or even neighbours can, and are willing to do the caring. This may not be the case due to other family commitments or frailties. Careful consultation, discussion and planning with the family can help ensure equality in the provision of health/care services. Many spouses or partners who are acting as carers are reluctant to accept help and can become gradually debilitated themselves. Approached sensitively, support to a partner, relative or friend may prevent a complete breakdown in their caring capability. For example, teaching how to wash and dress a dependent partner without undue strain can avoid or postpone the need for greater intervention.

Modesty

When caring for People it is important to be aware of their attitudes to their bodies and how they feel about someone else caring for them when they are most vulnerable. It is also important to understand the attitudes of their close family. Many of the People whom you will support may be of a different generation to you. In some cases they may not be happy to undress in front of another person; some may not even have allowed their partners to see them undress. To be expected to do so with a stranger could be very difficult for them to accept. If you need to help them move from their bed or chair for hygiene purposes, you should try to keep some kind of covering so that they can maintain their dignity. Many of us, however 'modern' we believe our attitudes to be, might not be happy to expose our bodies when we are feeling unwell and vulnerable. Many women and their families would find it unacceptable to have a male carer visiting a woman; this may be due to their personal attitudes or to cultural and religious beliefs. You should, therefore, discuss this with them when planning their care, as sometimes they may refuse services if they feel they have no choices about who their carers will be.

Language

You should encourage anyone whose understanding of English is limited to have an interpreter. Remember also that, for People whose mother tongue is not English but who have managed in English for much of their lives, the experience of illness might affect their command of the language. An interpreter must be totally aware of what information you require, as well as conveying the correct information to the Person you are assessing. An interpreter should ideally be a professional. A responsible family member may be used, but it must be borne in mind that they are not neutral and may try to convey what they think the Person *should* want rather than what they actually say, and this may not be because of self-interest. Young children should not be put into the position of asking intimate questions of their parent or grandparent. Once an assessment has been completed, there should be feedback with the help of the interpreter. Remember that many English words do not have direct translations into certain languages and therefore the accuracy and understanding of the interpretation should be checked. Many People may find it helpful to have a leaflet, in the appropriate language, detailing this information. Most Social Service Departments and Health Authorities have lists of people who are able to translate or interpret.

Making changes in the home

The philosophy behind care in the community is to emphasise the importance of enabling People to live as independently as possible in their own homes (DoH, 1995). Care and support is targeted to their requirements and preferences. The aim is to assess a Person's particular needs and to tailor services to meet those needs. This means that services must be flexible and will be offered by various providers in both the statutory and the independent sector. While this gives more choice to the Person, it does bring additional risks to carers working within the home environment. There needs to be liaison between agencies and care providers, and clear guidelines and procedures to ensure continuity and consistency of care. A good risk assessment and clear documentation of how care will be offered to a Person will help reduce risks to all concerned (see Chapter 3: Assessing Risks). There are several risk factors within a Person's home, and it is important to consider risks to the Person receiving care, the others who may live with them and the carer. It must be remembered that as a carer you are effectively a guest in a Person's home and therefore can not demand changes.

COMMON ENVIRONMENTAL PROBLEMS WORKING IN PEOPLE'S HOMES

Below are just some of the environmental problems which you may face:

- low, soft, old saggy double beds, often with restricted access and usually not on wheels
- divan beds
- marital beds which People are reluctant to change
- heavy furniture which is often unstable, heavily loaded and difficult to move
- small rooms with poor access and lack of space for easy movement
- loose rugs, and worn out carpets which become a tripping hazard
- wet floors which may be a slipping hazard

♦ trailing wires, telephone cables, lamp leads etc.

♦ general lighting is often poor and hazards may be missed

♦ electrical, heating or gas appliances may be dangerous

♦ clutter and belongings piled up on the floor often next to chairs and beds for easier access by the Person.

HELPING PEOPLE TO ACCEPT CHANGE

People are often reluctant to accept change, unless they can understand the problem and see the sense in the proposed solution. They may be especially reluctant if the change involves new equipment, which may feel intrusive and may present them with confirmation of their disability. Resistance to changes being introduced may also be due to fear of leaving the past behind, for example, if a spouse has recently died and there is a suggestion of changing the marital bed. A sensitive approach is required and careful negotiation towards change is vital. You must be clear about the reasons for the change and the benefits it will bring as well as being sympathetic to the Person's feelings. The involvement of a social worker or someone who can give time to discuss any fears can be a great help.

Examples

a.   A request to move a disabled man downstairs to a single bed was unacceptable to his wife. The risks of the man falling on top of the carer as she pushed him upstairs at night were unacceptable to the care staff. The wife was herself disabled but preferred to struggle and assist him upstairs at night rather than move him downstairs. The man was extremely breathless and had heart failure. After careful discussion with a social worker, occupational therapist and moving and handling adviser, the couple revealed that they had been separated during the war and had suffered a dreadful ordeal; since being reunited they had never spent a night apart. Eventually, through careful explanation and planning, stressing the safety of both the man and his wife, the bed was moved downstairs.

b. A man was terrified of being dropped or falling through the sling of a hoist. Following gentle explanation and encouragement, he now finds the use of the hoist a reassurance, as he does not experience any pain on transferring from one position to another.

c. Another man was happy to have a hoist introduced into his home but unfortunately his wife did not like the change and hid the slings. Following much persuasion she now appreciates the benefits to her husband and those caring for him, and both are now quite happy to have the hoist.

Source: District Nursing Team, Eastbourne and Community Health Care Trust

RESOURCES

Once People agree to changes, there may be a delay in the provision of equipment due to a lack of resources. There may be prolonged discussion over who will pay for equipment. Managers must bear in mind that during this delay People may be at risk and it may be necessary to take additional precautions. They may also be distressed by the delay. It is vital to ensure that risks are minimised and that carers and the People they are caring for are not being put in danger. For example:

- careful monitoring of deterioration in the situation
- more carers allocated in the short term
- rotate carers so that there is less repetition of difficult tasks
- avoid moving the Person; care for them *in situ*, i.e. in bed in the short term
- find alternative care while waiting for equipment e.g. respite care
- borrow equipment from medical loans departments.

It is better to be prepared and have a stock of small handling aids and hoists readily available. The argument over who pays will depend on the needs of the Person. If a nursing need is identified, then medical loans may provide equipment subject to the nursing input (NBPA, 1998). If the equipment is seen as an aid to daily living, funding for the change is available from local authorities but People will be means tested. In many cases there is joint funding. Although this offers a good solution it does result in delays during which People are at risk.

SUMMARY OF SUGGESTIONS TO IMPLEMENT CHANGES

1. Well planned discharges from hospital. Good liaison between Health and Social Service staff.

2. Channels of communication, for example, case conferences, home visits and care planned in advance of discharge.

3. All equipment installed prior to provision of care or as soon afterwards as possible.

4. Introduce changes sensitively but make it clear that carers are not permitted or prepared to take unnecessary risks; unless a safe system of work is in place the task will not be completed.

5. Ensure the Person and all family members are aware of the benefits of change and of the consequences of refusing the changes.

6. Involve a third person to negotiate if there are problems accepting change; social workers are particularly geared towards this role.

7. Shared loans stores are useful (Social Services and Health Services).

8. Ensure regular meetings and feedback involving all agencies participating in the care package.

9. Draw up shared risk assessments and keep them in the Person's home (see Chapter 3: Assessing Risks).

Key Points

♦ Respect the Person's individuality.

♦ Maintain good communications.

♦ Understand and address the needs of the family and other informal carers.

♦ Work to develop partnerships with family and other key people providing care.

♦ Be aware of cultural and religious differences.

♦ Allow People to be independent.

♦ Encourage People to return, as far as possible, to independent living.

♦ Ensure the caring environment is safe.

♦ Review the care needs on a regular basis, setting objectives and target dates.

A word about you

Caring for you as a carer is most important. It is very easy to give all your attention to the needs of the Person and their family, forgetting that your own health and safety are essential parts of the care equation. You should tell your manager if you have any concerns that a Person's needs may affect your safety, so that alternatives may be put into place. You should also tell your manager if a Person will not agree to changes in their home which will then affect how you are able to fulfil your role.

♦ Stay fit. If you are in good health you will be able to work more effectively.

♦ Stress, particularly emotional stress causes muscles to contract and this can be an important contributory factor when injuries occur. Chronically contracted muscles decrease the circulation of blood and oxygen, and can result in pain and atrophy. It is therefore important to be aware of and to practise some stress management techniques.

  ❖ Relaxation is not always at the top of the agenda when you are busy, but you should give thought to how you 'get away from the job'. For example, the use of relaxation tapes can allow you to focus away from a situation. This may enable you to review how you manage People and situations that you find difficult.

  ❖ Yoga, exercise at the gym, kicking a football around a field brisk walking and any form or aerobic exercise which will increase the flow of oxygen-rich blood through the body will be positive. This will enable you to cope more easily as well as giving you extra energy. In addition to these techniques, hobbies of any kind can help you to deal with stress.

Remember that one cannot always change the situation in which one find onerself. The experience of loss - of one's physical capacity, independence, partner or peers - is such a common feature of People's lives when they need care. Working as a carer, you are exposed to the feelings generated by these experiences of loss. They can be distressing and difficult to deal with. This can be compounded if carers themselves have similar problems of loss in their own lives. Changing the Person may not be possible, but you can work to change your attitude to them. Thinking about what you say and how you say it can have a profound effect on the situation and your attitude to what you are trying to achieve. Moreover, you must be prepared to discuss difficulties with your manager. Managers need to recognise this as a common focus in supervising their staff.

REFERENCES

Bannister, C., (1996). *Learning not to lift. Nursing Standard, 2 (2): 25-6.*

Department of Health (Social Services Inspectorate), (1995). *Caring for People at Home. HMSO, London*

Hempel, S., (1993). *Home Truths - Safe Handling of Patients in the Community and Problems Encountered. Nursing Times, 89 : 40-41.*

Holis, M., (1991). *Safer Lifting for Patient Care. Second edition. Blackwell Scientific Publications, Oxford.*

Kelly, J., (1996). *A Safer Passage: Mobility and Safety. How Nurses changed the environment to reduce falls for a patient with dementia. Nursing Times, 1(92) No. 4: 58-60.*

Lloyd, P., (1997). *Moving Patients. Community Nurse, 3(8):25-6.*

McGuire,T., Moody, J., Hanson, M., and Tigar,F., (1996). *A study of Clients' Attitudes towards Mechanical Aids. Nursing Standard, 11(5):35-8.*

Martin, J., Meltzer, H. and Elliott, D., (1998). *The Prevalence of Disabilties among Adults (1988). In: Survey of Disability in Great Britain, OPCS Report 1. HMSO, London.*

Meredith, B., (1995). *Community Care Handbook. Age Concern, England.*

Morgan, P., and Lawton, C., (1996). *Ethical Issues in Six Religious Traditions. Edinburgh Press, Edinburgh.*

National Back Pain Association (1998). *The Guide to the Handling of Patients, 4th Edition. National Back Pain Association in collaboration with the Royal College of Nursing, London.*

Royal College of Nursing, (1996). *Manual Handling Assessment in Hospitals and Community: An RCN Guide. RCN, London.*

Seymour, J., (1996). *Patient Handling - Safe Practice. Nursing Times, 92(32) : 46-8.*

Sinclair, I. et al, (1988). *Bridging Two Worlds: Social Work and the Elderly Living Alone. Avebury, Aldershot.*

Smale, G., and Tuson G., with Biehal, N., and Marsh, P., (1992). *Empowerment, Assessment, Care Management and the Skilled Worker. HMSO, London.*

Squires, A., and Arnold, E., (1991). *Multicultural Healthcare and Rehabilitation of Older People. Hodder and Stoughton, London.*

Thomas, S., (1996). *Safer Handling Campaign (Safe Patient Handling for Nurses and Carers including the RCN's recent campaign). Primary Care, 6(5) : 6.*

Tarling, C., (1992). *Handling Patients. Nursing Times, 10(88) : 38-40.*

6 Equipment: what's available and how do I use it?

Ron Steed & Clive Tracey

Introduction

There is a vast range of equipment available that can substantially restore People's independence and enable them to regain control of their daily living. In addition, equipment can eliminate or reduce the risk of injury to carers. Mechanical assistance involves the use of a range of aids. A sling hoist, for example, either powered or hand operated, can support the weight of the Person, leaving the carer free to control its positioning. Such aids can reduce risks but they do not always eliminate all risk. An element of 'manual handling' using bodily forces may still be needed to move a Person receiving care (NBPA, 1998).

If tasks involving 'manual handling' cannot be reasonably avoided, then the first question to ask is: 'Can I use equipment to eliminate or reduce the risk?' The Royal College of Nursing, in its 'Safer Handling Policy' (RCN, 1996), advocates the elimination of hazardous 'manual handling' in all but exceptional or life-threatening situations. To achieve this, the hierarchy below is helpful to follow as a general guide:

♦ independent movement - i.e. the Person moves by themselves

♦ provide equipment to assist independent movement - e.g. sliding board for moving from bed to wheelchair

♦ provide equipment to eliminate the task - e.g. mattress variator for sitting up in bed

♦ provide handling aids requiring minimal to moderate assistance by the carer - e.g. hoist or low friction rollers.

What equipment is available?

SUMMARY

Independent movement

> No equipment is needed. The People being cared for are physically and mentally capable of moving themselves.

Equipment to assist independence

In bed

- ♦ overhead hoist with access sling
- ♦ rope ladder
- ♦ mattress inclinator
- ♦ hand blocks
- ♦ monkey pole
- ♦ bed lever

Lateral transfer

- ♦ sliding board (bridging or transfer boards)

Standing/walking

- ♦ chair and bed raisers
- ♦ riser chair
- ♦ standing/walking aids

Equipment to eliminate the task

In bed

- ♦ electrically-mechanically - or hydraulically-operated bed
- ♦ mattress inclinator
- ♦ overhead hoist

Lateral transfer

- ♦ overhead hoist

Standing/walking

- hoist with specialised slings
- standing hoist

Equipment using minimal to moderate carer assistance

In bed

- low friction roller
- hand blocks
- overhead or mobile hoist
- handling sling (or strap)

Lateral transfer

- overhead or mobile hoist
- sliding board
- turning plate
- handling belt
- standing hoist

Standing/walking

- chair and bed raisers
- standing/walking aid
- handling belt
- riser chair
- hoist with specialised slings
- standing hoist

(See also Cassar, Costar & Tracey, 1998 for a survey of available equipment)

Equipment and its use

HOISTS

A correctly selected hoist can revolutionise a Person's lifestyle. It can facilitate dignity, comfort, safety and independence. The particular needs, size and weight of the Person should dictate the selection of a hoist. A note of caution: some people exceed the weight limits of various hoists and slings; when this happens an alternative, heavy-duty, hoist needs to be provided. It is essential in these circumstances that carers do not lift the Person without the aid of this hoist; this is extremely dangerous. If the Person is too heavy for a mechanical device, then they are too heavy for the more delicate human structure. Seek assistance from your manager or Manual Handling Adviser.

Overhead Tracking Hoist

An overhead tracking system can be a straight line, curved or X/Y system. One main advantage of these systems is that there are no storage problems since the whole system is attached to the ceiling or upper walls, or is mounted on high pillars. Single, straight or curved tracking systems (Fig. 6.1), can only lift the Person from a position directly under the track and this may limit their use. X/Y tracking systems (Fig. 6.2) consist of two parallel tracks fitted to both sides of the room with a moving section running between them. X/Y tracking systems are more flexible and a Person can be lifted from any point within the room, including over furniture (chairs, beds, etc.).

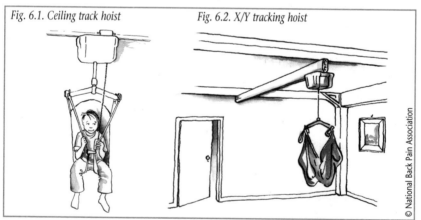

Fig. 6.1. Ceiling track hoist

Fig. 6.2. X/Y tracking hoist

© National Back Pain Association

Both types are electrically operated with a battery backup; movement along the track is either manually or electrically operated. A definite advantage with such systems is the vast height the hoist is able to lift and its ability to go to the floor without adjustment. These hoists may require permanent structural alterations that may limit their use within a Person's home, in nursing or residential homes. Many People with good levels of mobility may be able to transfer independently, providing they can fit the sling themselves. In this instance, an access sling is often advantageous (see below, page 82 (Toileting access sling)).

Mobile Hoists

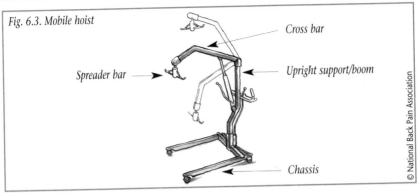

Fig. 6.3. Mobile hoist

Cross bar

Spreader bar →

Upright support/boom

© National Back Pain Association

Chassis

Sling Hoist

Mobile hoists (Fig. 6.3) allow transfer from one point to another anywhere, but they have the disadvantage of presenting storage problems and sometimes being incompatible with furniture in the home (see Chapter 5: The Person and the environment). A carer can shift a mobile hoist from one area to another by pushing it on its wheels (Note: it is not intended to transfer a Person from one area to another in this way). The hoist consists of a wheeled chassis, an upright support and a crossbar. The chassis may not be compatible with existing furniture, because it may not open widely enough to go around chairs, or may be too high to fit under beds etc. The chassis height is dictated by the wheel size. Larger wheels allow easier movement especially across deep pile carpets and uneven floors. For greater access around furniture, the width of the chassis may be controlled usually by lever or battery operation. The hoist's lifting range is governed by the length of the upright boom and crossbar. The range is particularly important when you need to lift onto special mattresses fitted to beds, and also if it is necessary to lift a Person who has fallen.

Mobile hoists lift directly under the crossbar and spreader bar. Brakes are not usually applied except in exceptional circumstances when the hoist is used on uneven surfaces or, following manufacturer's recommendations, when lifting a Person up from the floor. Refer to the manufacturer's instructions for specific hoists.

Lifting is achieved either by hydraulic hand pump, by winding a handle or by battery power. The hydraulic and handle-wind mechanisms require effort by the carer operating the hoist. Battery-powered hoists do not, but they do need to be recharged. Some battery-powered hoists have a two-battery system to reduce the likelihood of the hoist being left uncharged. Battery-powered hoists allow the Person to operate the hoist themselves and thus promote a greater level of independent movement.

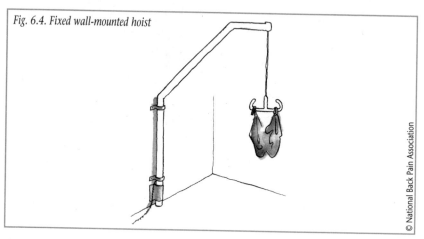

Fig. 6.4. Fixed wall-mounted hoist

© National Back Pain Association

Fixed and Wall Mounted Hoists

These types of hoist are securely fixed to the wall or floor; some may be moved from one fixed mounting to another (Fig.6.4). The length of the boom and crossbar dictate the range of movement. These may be electrically or battery operated and may allow independent movement as long as the Person can push themselves. They can be fitted into confined spaces where mobile hoists may not be able to fit. They can also be located behind furniture, which can overcome storage problems.

Slings for Hoists

Correct sling fitting will affect the level of comfort, function, independence and dignity that can be achieved for the Person and it will also help to overcome any unwillingness to use the hoist. Generally, the more material in the sling, the more support it will provide. A sling with less material is less supportive and requires more ability on the part of the Person being moved to support themselves using upper body strength. If a sling is incorrectly fitted, it may reinforce a negative attitude towards the use of a hoist or a refusal to be hoisted again.

How you fit slings depends on what you are going to do and your ability to fit them correctly. The position of the Person to be moved will also affect fitting, as will the furniture and environment (e.g. chairs that are too low or narrow, double beds, etc.).

All slings should be clearly identified by the manufacturer's label which should show:

♦ manufacturer's name and address

♦ hoists they were made for

♦ appropriate British Standards

♦ size

♦ weight limit.

General Purpose Sling (also known as Quick Fit sling) (Figs. 6.5 and 6.6)

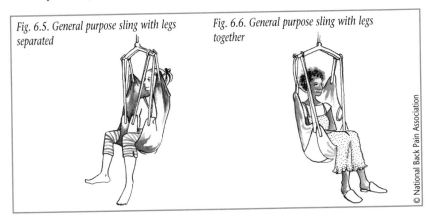

Fig. 6.5. General purpose sling with legs separated

Fig. 6.6. General purpose sling with legs together

© National Back Pain Association

This is a U-shaped piece of fabric with or without head support. It is generally the most comfortable type as body weight is evenly distributed over a large fabric area. You usually fit this sling while the Person is sitting or lying down. You can adjust the position and fixing of the leg bands to maximise dignity and comfort, and, if necessary, to allow access for cleaning perineal areas or so that the Person can use the toilet.

Hammock commode sling (Fig. 6.7)

This is a full-length rectangular sling with or without a commode opening. Pressure is distributed more widely over the fabric area. It is not as versatile or as easily fitted as General Purpose and Quick Fit slings.

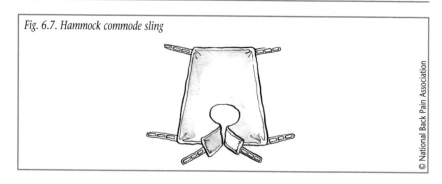

Fig. 6.7. Hammock commode sling

© National Back Pain Association

Amputee sling (Fig. 6.8.)

Slings are available which can accommodate People who have had either one or both legs amputated. These allow for greater support and comfort to the affected limb or stump while making the hole smaller.

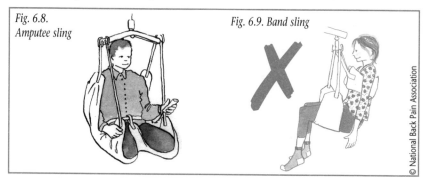

Fig. 6.8. Amputee sling

Fig. 6.9. Band sling

© National Back Pain Association

Band Slings (Fig. 6.9.)

Band slings are made from two narrow bands of fabric or hard vinyl-type material. One band is fitted under the thighs and the other around the back. However, following a Medical Devices Directorate Hazard Notice (Medical Devices Agency, 1994), these slings are not recommended for use as they can easily split apart when fitted, and may cause the Person to slip through the sling and fall.

Toileting access sling

These slings fit between the legs and around the chest and back allowing access to the Person's clothing and making using the toilet easier. You can be fit them with the Person in most positions, but slings from some manufacturers may require the Person to have control of the upper trunk of their body. These slings are generally the most appropriate when using overhead or fixed hoist systems to increase the Person's independence.

Bathing sling

Made from a mesh fabric, these slings allow water to drain quickly through the fabric so the sling dries quickly after use.

Stretcher sling (Fig. 6.10)

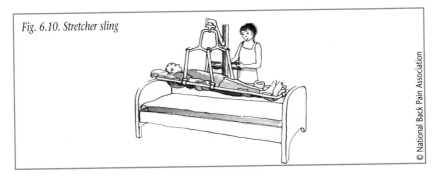

Fig. 6.10. Stretcher sling

© National Back Pain Association

These are specialised slings which allow a Person to be transported lying flat. They may be either full-length fabric, full-length rigid scoop frame or made up of a series of flexible bands which are inserted under the Person and attached to a frame that surrounds them. Not all hoists can accommodate these slings.

Walking harness sling (Figs. 6.11 and 6.12)

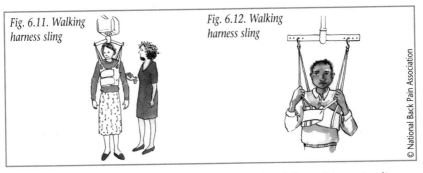

Fig. 6.11. Walking harness sling

Fig. 6.12. Walking harness sling

© National Back Pain Association

This is a specialised sling used to support People while walking, standing or dressing, and is especially useful during rehabilitation. It is used with an overhead tracking or mobile hoist designed specifically for these slings. It attaches around chest and the upper trunk and may have leg straps.

Specialised slings

Made to special order, these slings cater for specific needs that may not be met by the other standard slings. You may need specialised slings, if for example you are caring for a Person weighing more than 191 kgs (30 stones), or for People with fragile skin conditions, spinal or other physical abnormalities.

Standing / Toileting Hoist (Fig. 6.13)

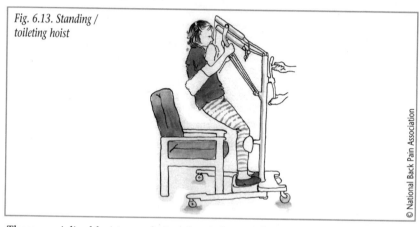

Fig. 6.13. Standing / toileting hoist

© National Back Pain Association

These specialised hoists are designed to help transfers from one point to another when the Person is in a seated position and being moved to another seated position (e.g. from sitting on the side of bed to the toilet or commode). They are useful for assisting with dressing, transfers or toileting, particularly for People who need support while standing. Many People prefer these hoists to a sling hoist because they allow them a greater degree of privacy, dignity and participation. For transfers, you should always use the transport sling or seat attachment so that the Person remains supported in a seated position throughout.

Most toileting hoists should be used for People who can partially weightbear through their legs and have arm strength. However, slings are available for some hoists of this type that allow them to be used with more dependent People. Individual assessment is essential, with much care being taken in the choice of slings.

Caution! These hoists will not suit everybody, and are not recommended for People with painful shoulders.

Equipment to assist independence

IN BED

Profiling beds (Figs. 6.14 and 6.15)

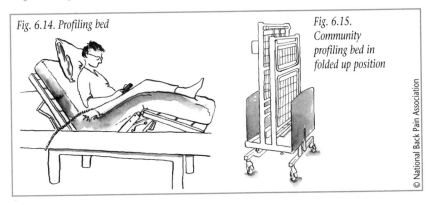

Fig. 6.14. Profiling bed

Fig. 6.15. Community profiling bed in folded up position

© National Back Pain Association

Their use greatly reduces the risk of injury to the carer through decreased handling, while electric beds greatly increase the independence of many People using them. Essentially they have the capability of converting from a flat-bedded platform into a combination of positions which are helpful for medical and comfort reasons. Profiling bed platforms come in either two, three or four sections. The choice of the platform positions can help prevent a Person slipping down in a bed, or decrease the number of times they need to be repositioned. With the back rest up, there is a tendency for the Person to slip down. Raising the knee or foot section slightly will help prevent this (Fig. 6.14). Newer models have a built-in automatic knee break.

All profiling beds are of variable height, operated either mechanically or electrically. The latter reduces the effort for the carer. However, many profiling beds designed for the nursing home or acute care areas cannot be disassembled and this makes delivery hazardous. There is now a range of electrically-operated profiling beds, at a reasonable price, designed for the community (Fig. 6.15). These beds allow the platform section to be dismantled into two, with the motors located on the head and footboard sections. The advantage of the community bed is that it can be delivered in four sections, each a manageable load and size, and assembled in the Person's home. They are not restricted to ground floor only installation, as is the case with the acute type of one-piece bed.

Overhead hoist

See above, page 78, this is used with an access sling and a toileting access sling.

Rope ladder (Fig. 6.16)

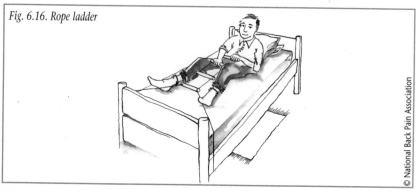

Fig. 6.16. Rope ladder

This enables a Person to sit themselves up by pulling along the rungs. Upper body strength is essential. The ladder must be attached securely to the bottom of the bed frame or legs. Some alternatives, which also allow independence, include grab rails, cot sides or side handles (available on newer beds) etc.

Leg lifting devices

These are for the Person who is unable to lift their legs up and onto the bed. They also remove the need for the carer to adopt a stooped posture. Leg lifting devices range from single rope-like devices (Fig. 6.17) to electrically- or battery-powered mechanisms. Some are inflatable air sacs (Fig. 6.18) that gently inflate and raise the legs, while others are mechanically operated.

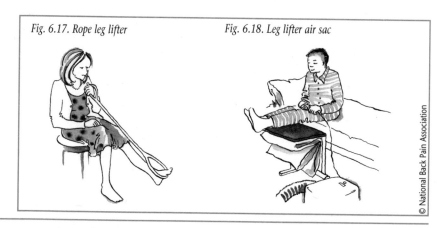

Fig. 6.17. Rope leg lifter

Fig. 6.18. Leg lifter air sac

Mattress inclinators (Figs. 6.19 and 6.20)

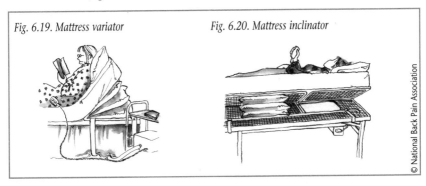

Fig. 6.19. Mattress variator

Fig. 6.20. Mattress inclinator

© National Back Pain Association

Designed to help the Person to sit up, these are fitted to ordinary divan beds under either the mattress or the pillows. Inclinators may be metal frames attached to mechanically driven arms that push/pull the metal frame up/down. Others are air sacs that are inflated by electrically-powered pumps. A limited number also assist the Person to turn from side to side. They can be noisy while inflating and deflating. An alternative is a profiling bed (see above, page 85).

Hand blocks (Figs. 6.21 and 6.22)

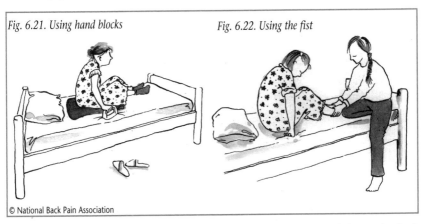

Fig. 6.21. Using hand blocks

Fig. 6.22. Using the fist

© National Back Pain Association

Hand blocks can be used to help a Person lift themselves up and down the bed independently. The Person must have upper body control and arm strength to one or both sides.

Caution! Hand blocks are solid and could cause damage or injury if they are thrown or dropped. It may be wise to use an alternative aid if the Person is confused or has a history of aggressive behaviour. Alternatives which fulfil the same purpose are: the Person makes a fist(s) or holds a rolled up towel in either or both hands and pushes into the mattress with the knees bent to assist pushing back.

Lifting poles (also known as monkey or trapeze poles) (Fig. 6.23)

These are used for lifting the top half of the body, assisting getting in and out of bed and for bridging so that bedpans and sliding sheets can be inserted. They are not to assist a Person to move up the bed.

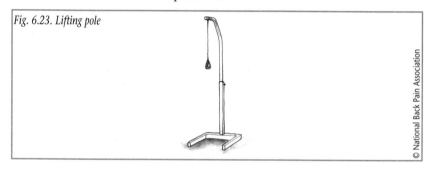

Fig. 6.23. Lifting pole

© National Back Pain Association

LATERAL TRANSFERS

Sliding boards (also known as bridging or transfer boards) (Fig. 6.24)

Rigid, semi-flexible boards or specially-designed low friction rollers with rods, these are used to bridge the gap between two surfaces (e.g. bed to wheelchair, wheelchair to commode, wheelchair to car seat etc.). The Person must have upper body and arm strength to shuffle their bottom across and move their legs sideways. When using these boards, People should be encouraged to lift their

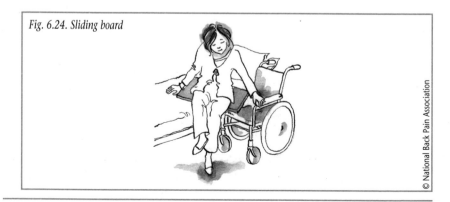

Fig. 6.24. Sliding board

© National Back Pain Association

bottoms rather than slide on the solid boards, to reduce friction. Some boards have a built-in transfer disc or low friction roller. Boards with built-in handles may help People to move, and are easier to pick up.

Caution! Low friction rollers should not be used on sliding boards as this may result in uncontrolled slipping and cause the Person to fall off the board onto the floor. If you are assisting then you should use a handling belt to improve your grip.

STANDING/WALKING

Chair and Bed Raisers

Blocks or extensions to increase the height of beds and chairs reduce the effort involved in rising from a low sitting position. They also lessen the amount of stooping for the carer. Two types are available:

♦ extension legs - fit around existing legs

♦ mechanical device - fitted under the bed to provide variable height.

Caution! Chair and bed raisers may make some furniture unstable. It may also be necessary to move or lift the furniture to insert the devices or extensions. Bed jacks are available to avoid lifting beds and should be part of any equipment stores. Homemade extensions may be unstable and may cause damage to the furniture.

Riser chairs (also known as ejector chairs) (Figs. 6.25 and 6.26)

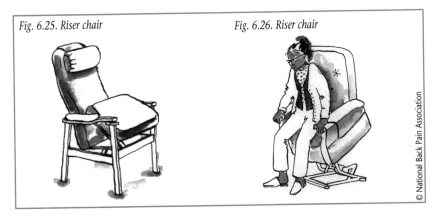

Fig. 6.25. Riser chair   Fig. 6.26. Riser chair

© National Back Pain Association

Mechanically or electrically operated to assist People with weak muscles or painful joints to stand, these work by raising the seat up and forward.

Caution! Mechanical seats must be adjusted for the Person's weight so that they do not eject too forcefully. Electrically-operated chairs have the advantage of a slow controlled rise.

Walking Aids

These are selected after specialised assessment by either a physiotherapist or occupational therapist and the Person who will use them. There are many different types of walking aid such as walking sticks and walking frames. (See Disabled Living Foundation, Hamilton Index (DLF, 1994)).

Equipment to eliminate the task

IN BED

Profiling Beds

Profiling beds can assist the Person to sit up, bend the knees or stand. With People who are more dependent, if the section under the knees is raised before the Person sits forward, this will help prevent any slipping down in the bed and reduce the amount of moving and handling by carers. Mechanically- and hydraulically-operated beds need to be operated by the carer, while electrically operated beds may be worked by the Person independently. There are many benefits to profiling beds. Some of the main benefits of the electrically-operated type are:

♦ increases independence as the Person can sit up or lie down without the carer's assistance

♦ greater freedom - People can move when necessary

♦ prevents slipping down the bed

♦ People who are more dependent may be moved by one carer

♦ may reduce the amount of time required to care for the Person and therefore have cost benefits

♦ reduces risk, especially when assisting heavier People.

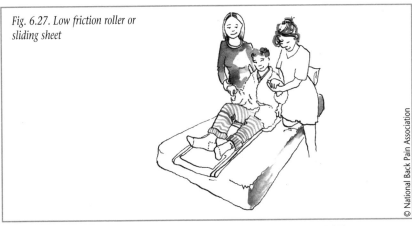

Fig. 6.27. Low friction roller or sliding sheet

© National Back Pain Association

Low friction rollers (also known as sliding sheets and sliding devices) (Fig. 6.27)

These are fabric sheets to move People without lifting or causing friction by sliding. There are two main types:

♦ roller, sleeping bag design

♦ flat sheet folded on itself or used with another sliding sheet.

Low friction rollers may or may not have handles, depending on the manufacturer. They are used to move People in a variety of ways:

♦ up and down in bed

♦ assist to get in and out of bed

♦ turn in bed

♦ reposition in a chair

♦ move from a confined space

♦ assist transfers from ambulance stretchers to bed etc.

They may allow People to move easily, unaided but with supervision, or they may require the carer to assist. In this case, the techniques used should be according to current best practice (see Chapter 8 sections 3, 4 and 8).

Caution! To avoid the risk of cross infection, low friction rollers used for one Person should not be used for anyone else. Carers should not use homemade improvisations. See Chapter 8 for home accessory items that may be used with low friction rollers (e.g. handling belt, towel, handling sling and bed linen).

Handling sling (also known as a handling strap)

A plastic, fabric or cushioned material band with hand holds, this is used by the carer to help a Person to sit forward in bed, slide up in bed with a low friction roller, or lean forward in a chair.

Caution! Never use two slings together as this will force you to lift the Person's full weight while in poor postures.

Turning plate (also known as a turning disc)

A turning plate of hard material or soft fabric design can be used to rotate a Person through 90 degrees. It may be used:

♦ independently after assessment for chair to chair/bed/commode/etc. transfers

♦ on car seats

♦ by carers to stand and rotate the Person

♦ to get in and out of bed.

Soft fabric turning plates can be used in a greater variety of settings than the hard material type.

Caution! People must be assessed, firstly because a turning plate narrows the base of support while standing (the feet are close together and the Person may therefore be unstable while standing), and secondly because they may cause disorientation when turning. Some turning plates with built-in roller bearings are harder to control during the turn, thus moving too quickly or in an uncontrolled manner, which can be frightening for the Person.

Handling Belt

This fabric or cushioned material belt is worn by the Person in order to give the carer a firmer handgrip. You can use it to help People stand, walk or transfer.

Caution! Handling belts are not a lifting device; they are merely supportive. Do not use the Person's own belt as their clothing may be pulled into the groin, the Person may be hurt by your knuckles or the belt loops ripped.

What to consider when purchasing equipment

TRAINING

All carers require sufficient training in the use and care of any piece of equipment they are expected to use, no matter how small or straightforward the item may appear. As a manager, you must consider how this training will be achieved before the equipment is bought. The training should be carried out by a competent person and follow local management guidelines. This training may be fitted into regular training sessions or additional ones may be required (see Chapter 4: Training).

CLEANING AND MAINTENANCE OF EQUIPMENT

You need to consider access to management cleaning and maintenance protocols. All equipment should be supplied with cleaning and maintenance information. Many hoists and small handling aids can be wiped down with soap and water or detergent, depending on local management policy and infection control protocols. Soft fabric handling aids, such as turning plates or low friction rollers, may be put into a washing machine. Before use, check all handling aids for damage, loose stitching and cleanliness.

INSURANCE

Equipment should be insured. The manufacturer insures all products that have not been altered and are used according to manufacturer's instructions. Defective or unsafe products that cause injury are the strict responsibility of the manufacturer (Consumer Protection Act and General Product Safety Regulations). If a product is altered (e.g. using a sling from one manufacturer on a hoist from a second manufacturer), you need to check with the hoist manufacturer that the sling is compatible and only then will they consider accepting liability. It is advisable to have this in writing. If not, check with your own insurers. Your insurers may not cover claims involving the use of broken or poorly maintained equipment. Insurers do not cover homemade equipment unless specifically negotiated with them.

MANUFACTURER'S INSTRUCTIONS

All equipment must now be accompanied by manufacturer's instructions (Medical Devices Agency, 1998). The instructions should highlight:

♦ the type of Person for whom the equipment is manufactured and any special considerations

♦ operation and training

- cleaning and care
- maintenance
- contact telephone number and support address.

SERVICING

Many pieces of mechanical and electrical equipment (e.g. hoists, beds) will need regular maintenance and servicing by appropriate skilled personnel to ensure they are in safe working order.

EASE OF USE

Before any equipment is purchased, it is good practice to try it out first. The reason for selecting the equipment, the People whom it is meant to support and the abilities of the staff who will operate it all need to be considered. It is pointless to purchase a large mobile sling hoist if the carer using it is not strong enough to push it across a carpeted floor.

CONSUMABLES

Certain equipment may require parts on a regular basis e.g. batteries, slings, etc. The cost of these parts should be considered and included in the routine maintenance programme if possible.

TRAINING ON USING EQUIPMENT

The employer has a legal obligation to provide adequate and up-to-date training on all equipment used. Carers must also take responsibility for informing managers if/when they feel they need more training or practice. Carers should not use equipment when they have not received adequate training. Training should be provided by someone with in-depth knowledge and experience of the equipment (see Chapter 4: Training).

STANDARDISATION

Managers should consider standardising the equipment provided. Standardisation decreases costs, reduces the time needed for training and allows carers to move from home to home in confidence, knowing the make of equipment they use will be the same in all situations. Slings for hoists can be shared, reducing the need for multiple sizes from different manufacturers.

ADVICE

Seek advice on the appropriate equipment from the manufacturer or an appropriately trained person such as a back care adviser or manual handling trainer. The advice should be based on a number of factors of which the most important are:

♦ individual assessment of the Person to be supported

♦ type of movement required

♦ the abilities of the Person and their carer

♦ the environment where the equipment is to be used.

DOMESTIC AIDS

Caution! Many domestic aids are unsafe to use. Homemade aids can pose a number of risks for the Person, their carer and the care manager:

♦ damage/harm the Person or the carer

♦ damage to other aids or furniture

♦ not tested for safety or weight limits

♦ not approved for the technique

♦ not insured

♦ not always compatible with existing equipment or techniques.

Environmental and external considerations

FURNITURE AND ENVIRONMENTAL CONSIDERATIONS

Assumptions

1. It is often assumed that all equipment can be used in all circumstances. This is not true. For instance, hoist legs may not open sufficiently wide to go around certain chairs or may be too high to go under a bed or chair. Consideration should be given to the space available, floor surface, width of doorways and height and size of furniture.

2. Fixed-height divan beds are common in People's homes. These may limit the range of safe techniques available to care staff and may determine the choice of equipment. If a bed is against a wall, a low friction roller may need to be used and, in rare instances left in place. [CAUTION: This is not recommended and will depend on the Person's mobility. If left in place, a

padded version may be needed (see Chapter 8: Some techniques)].

3. Equipment used in bathrooms or areas which may become wet must be suitable for that area. A sliding board with integral low friction roller can be used to help a Person who is not dressed to transfer from bath to wheelchair. Hoists, bath chairs and other electric- or battery-powered equipment should have waterproof controls to avoid electrical shocks.

4. Building alterations may be required for larger equipment such as specialised beds, hoists or overhead tracking hoists. The structure and suitability of the area must be considered with advice from a structural engineer (see also Chapter 5: The Person and the environment - Making changes to the home).

5. Carpet pile may affect the selection of castors on equipment. Equipment used in such areas should be tried out first for suitability before renting or buying.

Conclusion

BENEFITS

We have already said that appropriate equipment may restore a substantial amount of independence to a Person. In addition, equipment may reduce or eliminate the risk to care staff. The regulations require that the first question to be asked is whether risk can be eliminated. If not, then the requirement is to reduce the risk to the lowest level reasonably practicable (see Chapter 1: Legislation and responsibilities and Chapter 3: Assessing Risks). Using suitable equipment is a fundamental way of reducing risk, and the use of equipment should be considered before training. It may require the task to be redesigned to incorporate improved techniques.

The introduction of equipment:

- is safer and usually more comfortable for the Person and the carer

- promotes independence

- provides carers with alternative ways to move People with less risk to themselves.

RISKS

If you use equipment either poorly or inappropriately, it may not meet the Person's needs and may lead to injury. The consequences may be serious. Staff require training in the use of any equipment supplied, and must follow the manufacturer's instructions. Incorrect use may cause both the Person and the carer to feel unsafe or uncomfortable and may encourage reluctance or refusal to use appropriate equipment in the future.

There is a vast range of equipment but not all makes perform equally well. As a result, poor quality products may be purchased unwittingly. It has been known for poor quality equipment to be unsafe, for example, poor quality sliding devices have been known to rip!

Maintenance is often overlooked, leaving equipment, especially hoists, in a poor state of repair and, in the worst cases, unsafe. The cost of equipment, often perceived as a negative factor, should not become the prime consideration. Equipment must be purchased based on the individual assessment of needs and the tasks that have to be carried out to ensure that safe and high quality care is delivered.

REFERENCES

Cassar, S., Costar, S. and Tracey, C., (1998). Patient Handling Aids: prescribing guidelines. British Journal of Therapy and Rehabilitation, Vol. 5, No. 32.

Disabled Living Foundation, (1994). Handling People: Equipment, advice and information. Disabled Living Foundation, London.

Medical Devices Agency, (1994). Medical Devices Directorate Hazard (94) 18. Medical Devices Agency, London.

Medical Devices Agency, (1998). Medical Devices Directorate Hazard (98) 1. Medical Devices Agency, London.

National Back Pain Association, (1998). The Guide to the Handling of Patients, Fourth Edition. National Back Pain Association in collaboration with the Royal College of Nursing, London.

Royal College of Nursing, (1996). Introducing a Safer Patient Handling Policy. RCN, London.

7 Getting out and about

Kevin Tesh

Introduction

It is important for People to be able to get out of the house for exercise, stimulation and fresh air. For this to happen, certain equipment and facilities need to be in place to make the journey as easy as possible. Care providers have a legal responsibility to conduct risk assessments before care staff start to work with People in the community (see Chapters 1 and 3). In the care plan you need to include the assessment of risks associated with getting out and about. This must take account of the premises, the method of transfer and any equipment used, the Person's needs and the capabilities of the carers.

Using a wheelchair

You need to ensure that basic equipment, such as the wheelchair, is regularly maintained by the supplier (i.e. health services, social services or private agencies) so that:

♦ the brakes are working efficiently

♦ the wheels are running true and the tyres are inflated to the correct pressure

♦ all parts of the wheelchair are included and fitted correctly.

It is also important that the carer knows how to collapse and open out a wheelchair correctly and is trained in its use, for example using the tipping lever on the back of the wheelchair to assist with counter-levering it up a step or kerb. The weight of the carer relative to the weight of the Person is important so that the carer can comfortably push and manoeuvre the wheelchair without creating unacceptable loading on their back.

A powerpack can be fitted onto a wheelchair and this will reduce the effort required by the carer to push it. These powerpacks are particularly useful if the Person is heavy, or the distances to be covered are long or uphill. Make sure that the powerpack is adequately charged for any journey.

When planning a long outing, it is important to know how you will access toilet facilities. If this is going to be difficult, then you should see that the Person is protected by wearing high absorbency pads (in the case of a woman) or a condom/sheath with catheter and leg bag (in the case of a man); this will reduce any possible discomfort.

Getting out of the house

One of the biggest obstacles to getting out of the house is an uneven surface or steps which can be difficult for People whether on foot or in a wheelchair. Before you assist a Person to go out in either a wheelchair or on foot, it is imperative that you plan the route from the house to the road level to avoid uneven surfaces such as steps, gravel or stone paths. All these conditions can make it difficult to push a wheelchair, and present potential problems underfoot for someone who is unsteady on their feet. The route must be wide enough to accommodate a wheelchair or, if you are assisting a Person, sufficiently wide to allow two people to pass comfortably unimpeded by bushes, sheds etc. If the house has more than one exit, choose the most appropriate one.

Before starting, see that the route is clear and that all doors, gates etc. are open so that the Person can go in and out easily. Remove any household items from the doorway or porch if they block or restrict space on the route. Planning and clearing the route allows you to have both hands free to guide or support the Person if necessary.

Both you and the Person you are caring for need to be properly dressed for the weather conditions before you leave the house. Inadequate protective clothing in low temperatures makes any physical activity, even walking, more difficult and will make you both tire more easily. If your hands are cold, you will find moving and handling techniques may be more difficult to undertake. However, gloves can also restrict your manual dexterity, so be sure they fit properly. If the Person is walking, ensure that they wear comfortable and flat shoes.

The problem of steps can be overcome by providing an inclined ramp from the door of the house to road level which can fit over or replace the steps (Fig 7.1). Ramps are essential for wheelchair users and are preferable for People who are not confident when walking. If the ramp is temporary, it should be securely fixed so that it does not shift with use or in bad weather. It should be laid on solid foundations so that the floor surface does not move when people walk on it. The surface should be non-slip. For a Person who is more confident walking, you can have a handrail fitted down the side of the steps. This provides support when negotiating the steps and allows the Person to rest when going up or down.

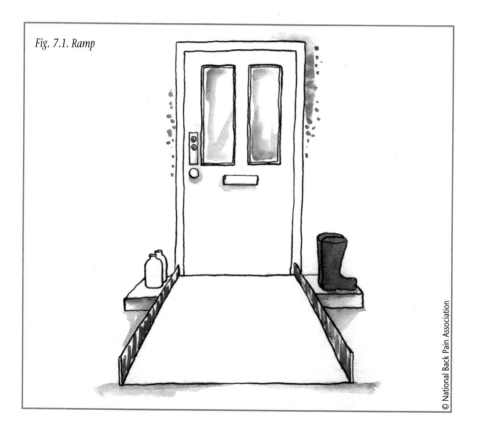

Fig. 7.1. Ramp

© National Back Pain Association

Getting into and out of a car

If a Person who uses a wheelchair needs to get into and out of a car, the car should be specially adapted. Equipment is available to enable the Person to remain in the wheelchair during the journey. There is a variety of adaptations including a car top hoist, ramps for entering the rear of the vehicle, swivelling car seats etc. (see Disabled Living Foundation, Hamilton Index (DLF, 1994)).

If a private car (or similar vehicle) has not been adapted, you need to consider some functional requirements first of all. These include:

- suitable storage capacity for wheelchair and other equipment (sliding sheet, soft or hard turning discs etc.)

- wide opening range of front and rear door with strong door stops

- easily adjustable seats

- fairly flat side rolls on seats to allow easy access to the vehicle (wedges can be used if the side rolls are deep)

- shallow footwell level relative to door sill to avoid excessive step height when getting into or out of the vehicle

- up-to-date disabled sticker openly displayed

- sign in the back of the vehicle to stop other motorists parking too close and obstructing access and working space to load and unload the wheelchair etc.

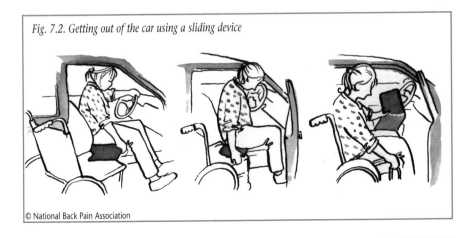

Fig. 7.2. Getting out of the car using a sliding device

© National Back Pain Association

Before you assist the Person to go from the house to the car, make sure the car is parked as close as possible to the exit you will use. Remember that you will need clear access to open the car doors and position the wheelchair alongside the car. This keeps the distance to walk or push the wheelchair to a minimum. If you need to load equipment such as a wheelchair into the boot, park the vehicle to allow plenty of working space at the back so that you can get to the boot easily and load the equipment safely without having to adopt poor postures. If possible, park the vehicle far enough away from the kerb so that the Person can place their feet on the road before getting into the vehicle. This effectively raises the height of the vehicle seat and reduces the distance the Person has to lower themselves when moving from standing to sitting. Similarly, when getting out of the vehicle the distance from the sitting to standing position is also minimised.

Open the door to its maximum before the Person gets into the car. Ideally, park the car with the passenger door alongside the kerb so that there is no danger from passing traffic. However, if this is impossible, remember that car doors can close unexpectedly if the vehicle is parked on a road with excessive camber and the Person is being assisted into the vehicle 'offside' or roadside i.e. towards the centre of the road. Strong winds or passing vehicles may also make the door suddenly close.

If the Person wants to sit in the front, move the front seat as far back as possible to give maximum legroom to swing their legs into the car. Conversely, if the Person wants to sit in the back, the front seat should be moved forward as far as possible. Once the seat has been adjusted, it should be fitted either with a sliding device or soft fabric turning disc (see Chapter 6: Equipment).

USE OF SLIDING DEVICES (Fig. 7.2)

Use sliding devices to reposition the Person back into a more upright position or to slide them into the centre of the seat. This eliminates the need to physically lift the Person; you can slide them to the correct position. If you perform this correctly, you will reduce the risk of injuring yourself. In order to gain a good grip it is best to have a sliding device with handles.

When pulling on the sliding device, be careful that you do not take up awkward postures and that the pulling is controlled so that you avoid sudden and unexpected movements. Particular postures to avoid include pulling with one arm while the back is twisted. For the most efficient pulling action with the least risk to you, you should position your body in line with the direction of pull and perform the pull with both hands.

For a Person sitting in the front seat, you should reposition the front seat forward, then sit on the rear seat and pull the sheet from each side of the backrest rearwards. The gap between the backrest and the central pillar housing the seat belt attachment may cause access problems with the left arm but you can usually solve this if the front seat is moved forwards once the Person is seated. You can adopt more suitable working postures when positioning a Person on the front seat using the approaches outlined above, so the front seat is the seat of preference when transporting a Person by car. Use of the front seat also allows more space for them to swing their legs into and out of the vehicle with the seat as far back as possible and the door fully open. If, however, the Person prefers to sit in the back seat, you must be particularly careful when repositioning them. It is difficult to apply a rearward pull on the sliding device without twisting because the backrest will prevent such a movement. If the Person has some lower leg strength, ask them to plant their feet on the floor and lightly push back so that the you can guide the sliding device back more easily. If this is not possible, two carers will need to be used, one on each side of the Person to move them back in the seat.

USE OF A SOFT TURNING DISC

A soft turning disc on the seat allows the Person to rotate fairly easily through 90° while seated. To assist a Person from a standing position into a vehicle, they should turn their back to the vehicle and you can assist them to sit down slowly on the side of the seat and onto the soft turning disc. Using the soft turning disc, the Person can be helped to turn their whole body to face the front of the vehicle. If the Person needs assistance to lift their feet, support their legs while they turn in the seat. Lift one leg into the car at a time, rather than trying to move both legs together. Alternatively you can use leg lifters if necessary. Follow the reverse procedure when helping a Person out of the vehicle.

For a Person able to stand, open the car door, position the wheelchair facing the front of the car, level with the central pillar and at road level if possible (Fig. 7.3a). Apply the wheelchair brakes. The Person stands, turns 90° and sits down in the car seat, making sure that they do not knock their head on the door frame. If the Person cannot stand, a sliding transfer from the wheelchair is carried out with the wheelchair positioned alongside the car but further forward, adjacent to the car seat (Fig. 7.3b). You can use a hard turning disc and/or transfer board for this transfer (see Fig. 7.2 and Chapter 8). The techniques described in Chapter 8 for a chair to chair transfer can be used. Once the Person is correctly seated in the vehicle, fit the seat belt and close the door. Follow the reverse procedure for getting a Person out of a vehicle into a wheelchair.

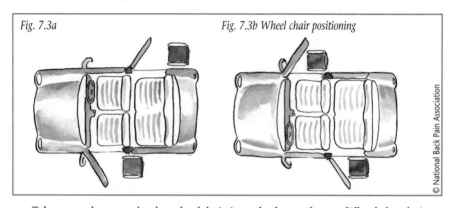

Fig. 7.3a   Fig. 7.3b Wheel chair positioning

© National Back Pain Association

Take care when you load a wheelchair into the boot of a car. Wheel the chair to the boot before folding it and lifting it into the boot. Ideally a wheelchair hoist should be fitted to the boot of the car. If not, it is important that you collapse the wheelchair properly and remove any wheelchair projections, such as front steering wheels or handles, or grasp them during the lift to avoid adopting awkward postures while putting the equipment into the boot. Remove accessories (e.g. foot and arm rests) before you lift the wheelchair, to decrease the weight you have to lift. You must make sure that there is sufficient storage space in the boot and lay a sheet over the boot floor so that you can bring the wheelchair closer to you when you lift it out of the boot. This is important if the boot area is large and the wheelchair is likely to move around during the journey. To lift the wheelchair, you should stand close to it and face the car boot. The wheelchair should be turned so that its heaviest side is closest to you when you lift it.

Group Outings

Transport can be provided for groups of People, for example for an outing from a residential home, by using specially adapted buses or minibuses. Access is provided by an automatic tail lift which is activated by a control panel located beside the tail lift or by a remote hand-held device. The tail lift is lowered to road level where the Person or carer wheels the chair onto the platform. On some tail lifts the wheelchair can be secured during the lift up into the minibus. Once secure, the carer stands back and activates the control to lift the Person up into the bus. Floor-mounted restraint devices must be fitted to the vehicle so that the wheelchair can be securely fixed in position for the duration of the journey.

Going into town

Currently there are few local bus services that are accessible to wheelchair users except in some cities, for example the Station Link bus in London. Most modern intercity trains can be accessed by wheelchair users provided arrangements are made in advance, as a special ramp is needed and spaces in carriages for wheelchairs are limited in number. Station staff will help wheelchair users board local trains but there is rarely any designated wheelchair space, so the Person has to transfer to a train seat for the duration of the journey. It is important to bear in mind that many stations are difficult to access and in some there are few or no staff on duty to help. Specialised taxis are available in some areas. Some local authorities run a shopmobility service where it is possible to hire either a manual or powered wheelchair/scooter. Dial-a-ride usually has a fixed drop-off and collection point near the shopmobility scheme.

You should be familiar with the layout of the town or city being visited. You should pay particular attention to the location of disabled parking places, wheelchair access toilets and lifts in department stores. In some larger cities, cycle maps are provided which show the gradients and any areas with steps. These can be a valuable source of information for planning a journey. This preparation will help to minimise unnecessary journeys and reduce the time for either pushing the Person in a wheelchair or assisting a Person who is walking. It is helpful if you know where there are any uneven pavements so that you can avoid unexpected movements when pushing a wheelchair. If possible, knowledge of any maintenance work on walkways or uneven pavements will help you avoid unnecessary additional strain or discomfort. Knowing the distribution of ramp kerbs around the town would also be helpful to reduce unnecessary journeys and make it easier to plan the shopping route.

Visiting the doctor or dentist

Most medical practices provide easy access for wheelchair users, with ramps or handrails along the sides of steps for People who are more confident on their feet. If a separate entrance is available for wheelchair users, it is helpful to see whether more convenient parking space is available closer to this entrance. When parking it is important to consider the need for sufficient space beside the passenger door to allow the Person to move or be assisted out of the vehicle. If you leave plenty of space between the car and other parked vehicles, it will be easier to access the boot if equipment needs to taken out. It is often better not to reverse into a space up against a wall as this may limit working space for getting items out of the boot.

Access to dentists' premises may present more problems because visits tend to be much less frequent than visits to a doctor's surgery and therefore the layout of the premises may not be as familiar. In addition, dentists' practices tend to be smaller and rarely provide dedicated parking spaces for patients. If visiting a dentist, it is well worth enquiring about access for wheelchair users or people who have difficulty negotiating steps etc. when making the appointment. Community dentists will often have facilities to make home visits if access to the surgery is too difficult.

REFERENCES

Disabled Living Foundation, (1994). Handling People: Equipment, advice and information. Disabled Living Foundation, London.

8 **Some techniques**

Sally Cassar, Joyce Cheney, Ron Steed

Introduction

The techniques described here should not be used without formal moving and handling training. Our aim, wherever possible, is to encourage the Person to participate usefully in any manoeuvre. The manual techniques described are to assist a Person only, and must always be preceded by an assessment of each situation to determine the level of assistance needed.

All manual handling tasks have an inherent risk and no amount of manual handling training or provision of equipment will eliminate all risk. Where a carer is put at significant risk assisting a Person to move, then mechanisation (e.g. the provision of a hoist) should be the priority. In all instances, follow the principles of the hierarchy of movement. These indicate an increasing level of risk to the carer:

♦ independent movement - first choice

♦ independent movement using small handling aids

♦ hoist or mechanical systems (e.g. profiling bed)

♦ two carers assisting a Person to move using small handling aids

♦ one carer assisting a Person to move using small handling aids - last choice.

Several techniques are considered unsafe. Please note that these unsafe techniques are highlighted in blue under each relevant section. A summary list of these unsafe techniques may be found on pages 166-174.

If you are going to use equipment, always ensure that the manufacturer's written instructions are accessible and that you follow them. Where appropriate, before carrying out moving and handling tasks, ensure the brakes and other safety features are in good working order and use them correctly. Whenever a carer is moving a Person in or around the bed, the carer needs to ensure the bed is at a suitable working height to allow good posture and the natural curves of the spine to be maintained (see Chapter 2: Principles of safer handling) and that the total combined weight of the carer(s) and the Person does not exceed the safe working load of the bed (you may need to check this with the manufacturer).

TERMINOLOGY AND ILLUSTRATIONS

For the purposes of this chapter the techniques can be carried out by either a male or female carer within their individual capabilities and limitations. If in doubt, don't do it! Seek help and advice. For clarity of description only, we have used the male pronoun (he) when referring to the Person and the female pronoun (she) when referring to the carer(s). In the illustrations, however, we have shown both and female People and carers.

When describing how the various techniques are to be carried out, we refer frequently to using the 'near' or 'far' hand or arm. When a carer has taken up position to begin a manoeuvre, her 'near' arm is the arm closest to the Person; her other arm is referred to as her 'far' arm. The same description is used to identify the specific limbs of the Person, for example, 'near' leg etc.

Techniques

1. Standing
2. Walking
3. Moving in bed
4. Sitting to edge of bed
5. Transfers
6. A falling or fallen Person
7. Getting up from the floor
8. Repositioning in chairs
9. Toileting
10. Special situations
11. Unsafe Techniques

1. Standing

Before assisting someone we must be clear about what we mean by standing. When it is noted that a Person 'Can stand with assistance' does this really mean: 'Two carers lift the Person into a standing position and the Person can then balance upright'; or 'The Person can stand upright but quickly loses balance and falls over'; or, alternatively, 'The Person is able to stand up and remain standing without falling, either with or without aids'?

Before asking a Person to stand, an assessment must be made to establish his strength, joint mobility and balance. The Person must be able to bear weight through both legs and have adequate strength to raise his body to a standing position. If lower limb muscles are weak, then equipment may be required to assist him to stand.

1.1. PREPARATION FOR STANDING

♦ Ensure the Person has adequate strength in his legs (see above) and is willing to stand.

♦ Fit the Person's footwear securely, ensuring the soles are non-slip.

♦ Clear the area of work and prepare the destination.

♦ Ensure all walking aids are close at hand and ready for use.

♦ Wherever possible ask the Person to push down on a stable surface (bed lever, chair arm) to assist himself to stand rather than holding onto you.

♦ Never let the Person push or pull up on a walking aid designed solely for support when standing (e.g. walking frame).

1.1.a. Positioning prior to standing from chair/toilet/commode/bed/etc

♦ Ask the Person to shuffle or rock on his bottom to the front of the chair (N.B. positioning in this way is appropriate prior to standing either with or without assistance). If assistance is required then follow the technique described in 8.3 (below), except that you move the Person forwards instead of backwards on the seat.

♦ Check the Person's feet are flat on the floor, hip distance apart and not tucked under the chair. It may be helpful to have him position one foot slightly forward of the other.

♦ Ask the Person to lean forward so he has a 'nose over toes' position.

♦ Gentle rocking of a Person forwards and backwards sometimes helps build momentum for the move.

♦ Ask the Person to push up on the arms of the chair into a standing position. As he stands, ask him to look up and ahead, not at the floor.

1.2. STANDING WITHOUT ASSISTANCE

Once the preparation is complete the Person may only need verbal prompting to stand. Standing can also be made easier by making changes to the chair (see Chapter 6: Equipment). If the Person is sitting on a low surface the carer cannot avoid adopting a poor posture if she is physically assisting with the stand. Independent standing from a low surface may also be more difficult for the Person himself.

1.2.a. Independent standing from a chair:

- The chair height should be such that a Person can sit down with his feet on the floor and thighs level, one foot slightly in front of the other, unless a footstool is required.

- The seat should be firm and the back rest should provide support for the seated Person. A lumbar cushion placed in the back of the chair may offer additional support and will bring the Person closer to the front of the chair.

- The arm rest should be well forward, at least to the level of the front of the chair. A padded arm rest is more comfortable for the Person to use for pushing up and assisting to stand.

- There should be space underneath the chair and at its sides if a carer is to assist a Person to stand.

- Ensure any footstool or walking aid is not in a hazardous position.

- Consider powered riser chairs and self-riser cushions to assist the Person to stand himself (see Chapter 6: Equipment).

1.2.b. Sitting down

- Ensure the Person can feel the front of the chair on the back of one leg or one of his knees.

- Ask him to reach down and touch the arm rests.

- The Person leans forward (nose over toes).

- The Person bends his hips and knees, at the same time sticking his bottom out towards the back of the chair while sitting down.

1.2.c. Independent standing from a bed with equipment

- The preparation is the same as independently standing from a chair (1.2.a).

- Bed levers or bed blocks may be useful in providing a more stable surface than the mattress (figs 8.1 and 8.2).

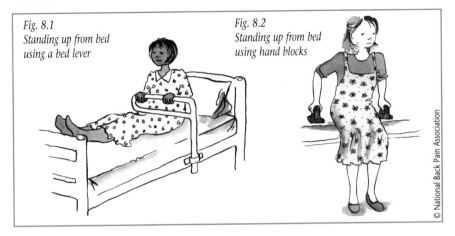

Fig. 8.1
Standing up from bed
using a bed lever

Fig. 8.2
Standing up from bed
using hand blocks

© National Back Pain Association

♦ If a carer is present and the Person is in a height-adjustable bed, the carer could raise the bed as the Person stands, thus facilitating the manoeuvre.

1.2.d. Assisting to stand using a standing prop

A standing prop could be used if a Person: has difficulty rising to a standing position but can weightbear, has trunk and upper body control and enough strength to pull himself up if holding onto something secure, is not confused and will follow simple instructions. A standing prop (Fig. 8.3) consists of a fixed or turning platform on which the Person places his feet, and often a knee plate joined to a height-adjustable handlebar. The carer must put her foot on the brake as the Person pulls up into a standing position. If the device has a turning plate, the carer can then gently turn the Person on the turning plate in the direction required. This aid has the advantage that, not only does the Person stand up using their own strength, but once standing it gives him a stable surface to hold. This will assist when adjusting clothing for toileting, or simply when moving from bed to chair.

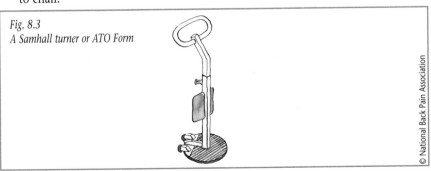

Fig. 8.3
A Samhall turner or ATO Form

© National Back Pain Association

Do not allow a Person to use walking aids to assist to stand, as they are designed to help with walking but may be unstable if used to stand up.

1.2.e. Assisting to stand using a standing hoist

A standing hoist (Fig. 8.4) could be used (see Chapter 6: Equipment) if a Person has difficulty rising to a standing position but: can weightbear, has trunk and upper body control but not enough strength to pull themselves up, is not confused and will follow simple instructions.

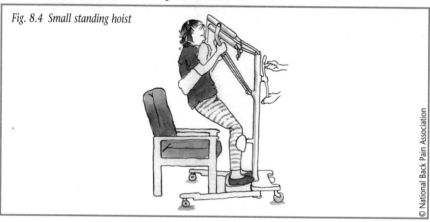

Fig. 8.4 Small standing hoist

© National Back Pain Association

The Person should be able to hold onto the hoist arms while placing his feet on the foot plate with knees resting against the knee-plate. It is important to position the sling well down the Person's back to avoid it riding up under the axilla (armpits). As the hoist rises it pulls the Person into a standing position. Once the sling is positioned it then raises the Person. If the sling slips up despite careful positioning, it could be that the Person is weightbearing insufficiently and a standing hoist is not suitable. Slippery clothing (nylon, satin, etc.) may also cause the sling to slip upwards.

1.3. STANDING WITH ASSISTANCE

Several methods can be used if more than verbal prompting is required to assist a Person to stand. Before starting any of these manoeuvres ensure the following:

♦ there is adequate access around the chair/seat to perform the techniques

♦ whenever possible ask the Person to push up on a stable surface rather than on a carer

♦ the carer should stand at the side of the Person facing the direction of travel with her feet apart and knees slightly bent

♦ the carer should be on the Person's weaker side.

1.3.a. Hand holds

Some carers feel more in control if they take the Person's hand. The handhold should be a palm-to-palm grip with the carer standing close (Figs. 8.5 and 8.6). The choice of interlocking thumbs or not will depend on any medical condition the Person may have (e.g. rheumatoid arthritis affecting the hands) and whether he likes to let go or not! If the Person is known to push or grab on the carer's hand, then it may be appropriate to use alternative approaches (e.g. chair arm or the Person's own leg just above the knee).

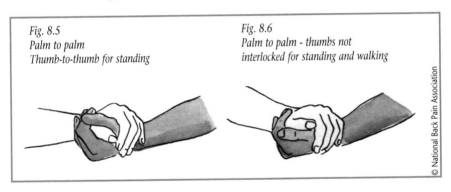

Fig. 8.5
Palm to palm
Thumb-to-thumb for standing

Fig. 8.6
Palm to palm - thumbs not
interlocked for standing and walking

© National Back Pain Association

1.3.b. Standing with assistance

This may be carried out by one or two carers depending on the Person's assessment.

Encourage the Person to push on a stable surface rather than on the carer.

♦ The Person is assisted to the front of the chair by shuffling forward or the carer may assist (Fig. 8.7).

♦ The carer must always be close to the Person if they are providing physical assistance to stand.

♦ The Person is brought into the 'nose over toes' position, that is, he leans forward (Fig. 8.7).

♦ The carer's far arm holds his hand palm to palm (with/without thumbs hooked), with the Person's forearm held level. (A palm-to-palm hold is not always possible and the carer may have to support at the Person's elbow (Fig. 8.8).

♦ The carer places her near arm around the Person's waist (Figs. 8.7 and 8.8).

♦ If possible, fit a handling belt to improve the carer's grip (Fig. 8.7, 8.8 and 8.9).

♦ Ask the Person to gently push down on the carer's palm as he stands up (Fig. 8.9).

♦ If there is only one carer and the Person has a history of not letting go, then ask him to push on the chair arm or push down on his knee (Fig. 8.10).

♦ The carer transfers her weight from her back leg to the front leg and moves with the Person as he stands, staying close all the time.

♦ Give clear commands of 'Ready, Steady, Stand'while simultaneously using gentle rocking motions.

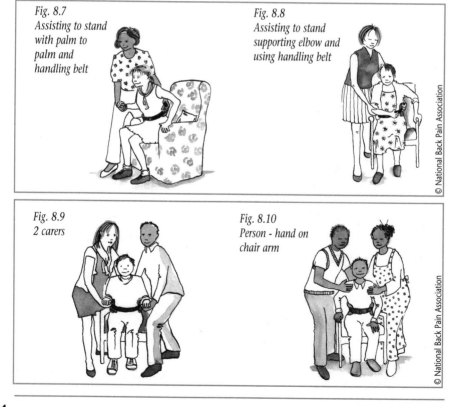

Fig. 8.7
Assisting to stand with palm to palm and handling belt

Fig. 8.8
Assisting to stand supporting elbow and using handling belt

© National Back Pain Association

Fig. 8.9
2 carers

Fig. 8.10
Person - hand on chair arm

© National Back Pain Association

♦ On the word 'Stand' during the forward rocking phase, the Person gently pushes down on the carer's palm as he stands. N.B. If the Person is putting a lot of weight on the carer's palm, this could indicate that his legs are not strong enough to raise him to a stand. At this point, reassess the suitability of a manual technique.

Once in a standing position, give walking aids if required (e.g. walking frame).

Certain techniques must be avoided. These include techniques that require the carer to stand in front of the Person, use the axilla (armpit), or grip the upper arm. (See 1.4 Unsafe Techniques.)

Standing with assistance in a restricted space

If there is restricted space or limited access at the side of the seat and it is not possible to create more space, then a handling belt must be fitted (Fig. 8.11). The carer adopts an upright stance in a slightly more forward position and grasps the belt at the side of the Person rather than at the back. This is a useful technique if a Person's foot needs to be stopped from slipping forwards or when standing from a bed. The carer will need to transfer her body weight sideways from rear foot to forward foot during this stand.

Fig. 8.11
Assisting to stand
from a chair in
restricted space/
poor access

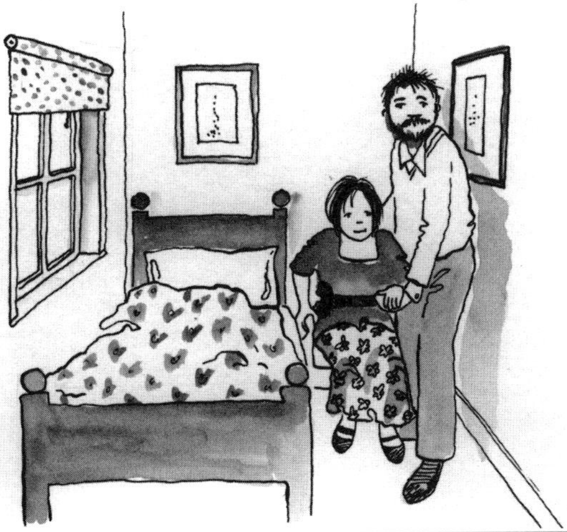

© National Back Pain Association

The movement described in 1.3.b. is used in reverse. It is important to make sure the Person can feel the chair is in position. Where possible ask him to reach down to the arm rests and lower himself to the seat. If there are two carers, it may be useful to cross arms at the back of the Person's hip or the handling belt. This will enable the carers to get closer and allow the Person to feel more secure. If a carer is assisting a Person to sit (or stand), it is important that she is in an unobstructed position and can move freely with the Person to avoid any sudden jerky movements or reaching and twisting movements. One or two carers can carry out this technique for Standing to Sitting and Sitting to Standing depending on the Person's assessment (Figs. 8.9 and 8.10).

1.4. UNSAFE TECHNIQUES (See also section 11 below)

⊗ UNSAFE TECHNIQUE - STANDING DIRECTLY IN FRONT OF THE PERSON

⊗ UNSAFE TECHNIQUE - UNDERARM DRAG OR ANY VERSION OF IT

⊗ UNSAFE TECHNIQUE - AUSTRALIAN / SHOULDER LIFT

⊗ UNSAFE TECHNIQUE - USING LINEN SHEETS TO LIFT OR DRAG

⊗ UNSAFE TECHNIQUE - PIVOT TRANSFER / BEAR HUG / STANDING TRANSFER

2 Walking

Prior to walking, consider the following points:

♦ Is the Person able to weightbear and move his feet without needing the carer to push or pull him forward in any way?

♦ Are both the carer and the Person wearing appropriate footwear?

♦ Is the Person well oriented, especially if it is night time?

♦ Is the planned route clear and have you considered equipment (e.g. catheters)?

♦ Have you made preparations for a Person who may be unsteady or recently inactive (e.g. extra carer, wheelchair behind the Person)?

♦ Can you rule out any other considerations that may increase the stress of walking (e.g. an urgent need for the commode)?

If the answer is NO to any of the above then you should reconsider the safety of this Person walking.

2.1 WALKING WITHOUT ASSISTANCE

2.1.a. Independent walking

The carer may use verbal prompting to encourage the Person to walk without the need for physical assistance.

2.1.b. Independent using walking aids

You can consider aids such as a walking stick/walking frame/crutches or the use of handrails.

- The use of walking aids may reduce the need for manual assistance.

- Any walking aids should be the appropriate height for the Person. This is usually assessed by a physiotherapist or occupational therapist.

- Consider safety features and ensure they are fitted if appropriate (e.g. rubber ferrules fitted to the end of the stick).

Don't use walking aids to assist a Person to stand. Don't allow the Person to hold onto them or push up from a chair onto them. Instead assist the Person to stand (see 1.4. above), then place the walking aid with him. (Exceptions to this may include the use of a tripod under guidance of a therapist.)

2.1.c. Mechanical assistance

A variety of hoists and walking systems are available (see Chapter 6: Equipment).

2.2. WALKING WITH MANUAL ASSISTANCE

2.2.a. Walking a Person who is unpredictable

Unpredictability is a common problem found frequently, for example, when caring for people who have dementia. 'Dementia' is a cognitive* disorder (Campbell, 1996). As a result of the unpredictability associated with this condition, one day a Person may walk unaided while the following day he may unexpectedly choose to sit on the floor. An unsafe and unnecessary method frequently used by carers is to lead the Person by the hand. If the Person decides to sit on the floor or suddenly change direction, the carer can be dragged along. If the Person does not need support, don't hold and/or lead them.

If the Person is familiar with the carer, his anxiety may be less and he may be better able to co-operate. This will reduce the risks to the carer. The important thing to bear in mind is that the Community Care Act (1990) allows the Person to take risks. A Person with dementia has this right so long as they do not put others at risk (see Chapter 5: The person and the environment).

2.2.b. Two carers

Always use a handling belt when a firmer grip is required (e.g. when a Person is wearing slippery clothing).

- Each carer puts her far hand into the appropriate hand hold with the Person (see Palm-to-Palm Grip 1.3.a) and holds his hand and forearm level at approximately his hip height (not too far up or down).

- With the near hand, each carer grips the handling belt.

- It may be useful for the carers to cross arms over the Person's back (Fig. 8.9).

- The carers should not thread their hands through belt loops but instead securely grip the loops.

- The carers position their hips just behind the Person but remaining close, with their feet apart in a good base of support.

- If a handling belt is not appropriate (e.g. a Person with abdominal problems), position as above but the carers' near hands now cross over the Person's back and are positioned at waist or hip level.

- The carers position themselves close to, but slightly behind the Person.

2.2.c. One carer

A handling belt is still the preferred option.

- The carer holds and positions as 2.2.b above.

- If a handling belt is appropriate, position handling belt as above.

- If a handling belt is inappropriate, position the carer's near hand on the Person's far hip.

2.3 UNSAFE TECHNIQUES (See also section 11 below)

- ✪ UNSAFE TECHNIQUE - PUSHING THE PERSON'S FEET FORWARD BY THE CARER USING HER FOOT

- ✪ UNSAFE TECHNIQUE - WALKING A PERSON WITH HISTORY OF FREQUENT FALLS

- ✪ UNSAFE TECHNIQUE - BEAR HUG / STANDING TRANSFER

- ✪ UNSAFE TECHNIQUE - UNDERARM DRAG LIFT

- ✪ UNSAFE TECHNIQUE - MANUAL LIFT FOR THOSE PEOPLE UNABLE TO TAKE THEIR OWN WEIGHT

3 Moving up in bed

3.1. ROLLING IN BED WITHOUT ASSISTANCE

3.1.a. Independent Rolling (Fig. 8.12)

Using verbal prompting, the carer should encourage the Person to turn towards her while giving the following instructions:

- ♦ turn head in the direction of the turn

- ♦ move his near arm either away from his side or lift and position the arm and hand onto the pillow or place it across the chest

- ♦ the Person places his far hand across his chest or holds onto the edge of mattress/bed in the direction of turn

- ♦ the Person flexes his far knee

- ♦ the Person rolls/pulls himself onto his side by pushing on the foot furthest away from the carer to assist.

3.1.b. Using grab rails, bed rails, bed lever, etc.

Using verbal prompting, the carer should encourage the Person to turn towards her while giving the following instructions:

- ♦ turn head in the direction of the turn

- ♦ move arm closest to the carer either away from the Person's side or lift and position the arm and hand onto the pillow

◆ place the hand furthest away from the carer across the Person's chest and he holds firmly onto the grab rail/bed rail/bed lever

◆ the Person flexes the knee furthest away from the carer

◆ the Person pulls/rolls himself onto the side nearest the carer and pushes on the right foot to assist.

3.2. ROLLING IN BED WITH ASSISTANCE

3.2.a. Two carers manually assisting a Person to roll without equipment

Raise the bed to the best working height for the shorter of the two carers. Both carers position themselves on the same side of the bed in the direction of travel. Carer One, at the head of bed, leads the manoeuvre and gives verbal commands clearly so that both the Person and Carer Two can hear. Using verbal prompting, the carer encourages the Person to turn his head, reposition his arms and bend his far knee. If the Person is unable to assist then:

◆ Carer One turns the Person's head in the direction of the turn, then moves the arm closest to the carer either away from the Person's side or lifts and positions the arm and hand onto the pillow. After positioning her own knee on the bed to reduce stretching, she positions the Person's far hand across his chest.

◆ After positioning her knee on the bed to reduce stretching, Carer Two simultaneously flexes the Person's far knee, then moves up the bed closer to Carer One (if the Person is unable to bend his knee, then cross his ankles).

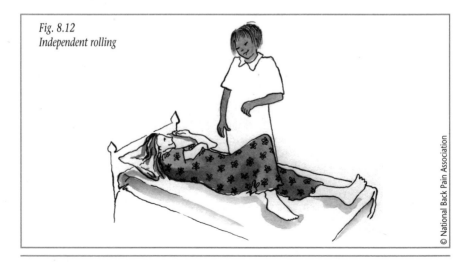

Fig. 8.12
Independent rolling

© National Back Pain Association

120

- Carer One positions one hand behind the Person's scapula (shoulder blade) and the other on his hip.

- Carer Two places one hand on the Person's hip, finding a space without crossing over Carer One's hand, then places one hand behind the Person's flexed knee (N.B. do not use the Person's flexed knee as a lever).

- Carer One clearly says 'Ready, Steady, Roll' and on the word 'Roll' both carers turn the Person onto his side towards them as they transfer their weight backwards, removing their knees from the bed but ensuring they do not step away from the bed. If they do so, the Person may feel he is rolling onto the floor and resist during the final stages of the manoeuvre.

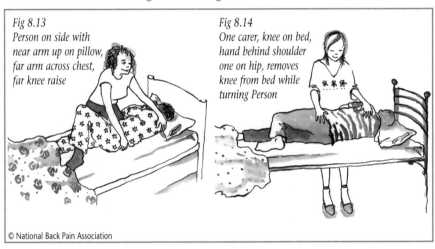

Fig 8.13
Person on side with near arm up on pillow, far arm across chest, far knee raise

Fig 8.14
One carer, knee on bed, hand behind shoulder one on hip, removes knee from bed while turning Person

© National Back Pain Association

N.B. If the Person has had a hip replacement recently, then bend his knee and avoid crossing his ankles.

3.2.b. One carer manually assisting a Person to turn/roll without equipment

Prior assessment must determine whether the Person to be turned is within the carer's safe capabilities.

- Raise the bed to optimal working height for the carer. The carer positions herself on the same side of the bed as the direction of travel.

- The carer gives verbal commands clearly so that the Person can hear and participate if possible.

- The carer turns the Person's head in the direction of the turn, then moves the arm closest to her either away from his side or lifts and positions his arm and hand onto the pillow. After positioning her own knee on the bed to reduce stretching, she positions the Person's hand that is furthest away from her across his chest (Fig. 8.13).

♦ The carer then moves down the bed, with her knee still on the bed to reduce stretching, and flexes the Person's far knee (Fig. 8.13) The carer then moves back up the bed placing her knee on the bed level with the Person's chest.

♦ The carer positions one hand behind the Person's scapula (shoulder blade) and the other on his hip (Fig. 8.14) with her elbow resting on his flexed knee if this is comfortable (N.B. do not use the Person's flexed knee as a lever).

♦ The carer clearly says 'Ready, Steady, Roll' (loudly enough for the Person to hear and participate) and, on the word 'Roll', turns the Person onto his side towards her as she transfers her weight backwards removing her knee from the bed but ensuring she does not step away from the bed. If she does so the Person may feel he is rolling onto the floor and resist during the final stages of the manoeuvre.

3.2.c. Padded turning sheet

This is a full bed-length sheet made of padded low-friction fabric which remains permanently underneath the Person, between the mattress and the bottom sheet. It is used specifically for turning a Person onto his side and is especially useful for someone who needs frequent turns with minimal disruption (e.g. hourly turns during the night). It can be used by one or two carers depending on the weight of the Person and the individual carer's capabilities. It is important to explain to the Person what is happening and the sequence in which it will occur.

For the initial placement of the padded turning sheet by two carers: if a hoist is available the Person can be lifted up, the padded turning sheet positioned on the bed and the Person returned to bed; if no hoist is available then, with the Person lying on his back, proceed as follows:

♦ The bed is raised to optimal working height for the carers who take up position one on either side of the bed.

♦ Carer One turns the Person onto his side towards her as noted in 3.1.b. above.

♦ Carer Two, positioned on the other side of the bed, places the padded turning sheet onto the mattress behind the Person in a similar way to changing a bed sheet.

- The Person is rolled flat onto his back then turned towards Carer Two, using the technique noted in 3.1.b. above.

- Carer One straightens out the padded turning sheet and returns the Person flat onto his back.

- The Person should now be in the centre of the bed with equal portions of the padded turning sheet on either side underneath him.

- Carer One positions the Person's head in the direction of the turn.

- Carer One positions the Person's near hand/arm away from his body or onto the pillow so he does not roll onto it.

- If bed rails are fitted, then Carer One raises the bed rail at the side of the direction of travel and joins Carer Two on the other side of the bed.

- If there are no bed rails, then Carer One remains on the side opposite the direction of travel.

- Carer Two flexes the Person's near knee.

- Carer One (or both if they are on the same side of the bed) firmly grasps the strong linen top sheet that is on top of the padded turning sheet, establishing a good base of support with her feet, and, on 'Ready, Steady, Turn', steps back while simultaneously pulling the strong linen top sheet slightly upwards. This backward and slightly upwards motion turns the Person onto his side (Fig. 8.15).

- The padded turning sheet is left in place and the bed sheet tucked in with creases removed (this will help prevent accidental slipping of the Person under the bed rails).

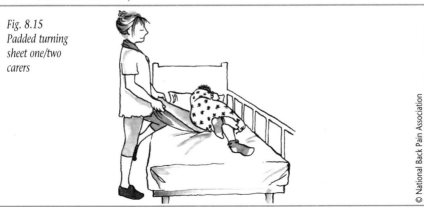

*Fig. 8.15
Padded turning
sheet one/two
carers*

♦ Place pillows behind the Person and between his knees for support. Roll the Person back onto the pillows at a 30 degree tilt (best practice to help reduce the risk of pressure sores). Do not position the pillows near his sacrum or any other bony prominence.

♦ Take care as too forceful a turn on a turning sheet may cause the Person to roll into the bed rail.

NOTE: A well-controlled use of this technique will help to ensure the Person is not accidentally rolled onto the floor nor frightened by too quick a movement.

3.2.d. Low friction rollers (sliding devices)

The low friction roller(s) are placed temporarily under the Person and should extend from the Person's shoulders beyond his buttocks. They are especially useful for turning a Person when a number of turns are involved (e.g. bed baths requiring multiple turns). The rollers are removed when the turns are completed. They can be used by one or two carers depending on the weight of the Person and the individual carer's capabilities. It is important to explain to the Person what is happening and the sequence in which it will occur.

Following risk assessment, a smaller Person may be turned by one carer. If only one carer is needed then raise the bed rail on the far side of the bed in the direction of the turn for the turn.

For initial placement of the low friction rollers by two carers, the Person should be lying on his back, then proceed as follows:

♦ Raise the bed to optimal working height for the carers (ideally hip height of the shortest carer) and they take up position one on either side of the bed.

♦ Carer One turns the Person onto his side towards her as noted in 3.1.b. above.

♦ Carer Two, positioned on the other side of the bed, places the low friction roller onto the mattress behind the Person, in similar way to changing a bed sheet, by rolling/folding half of the roller(s) and positioning it along the length of the Person (if using three small rollers then position one at head and shoulders, one at hip and one at heels) with open ends towards either side of the bed thus forming a continuous roll.

♦ Roll the Person flat onto his back. Carer One reaches underneath him and straightens out the roller(s) (N.B. if working alone do not reach over and under the Person but walk around to the other side of the bed to straighten out the roller(s).

- The Person should now be in the centre of the bed with equal portions of the roller(s) on either side underneath him.

- Carer One positions the Person's head in the direction of the turn.

- Carer One positions the Person's near hand/arm away from him or onto the pillow so he does not roll onto it.

- Carer One raises the bed rail at the side of the direction of travel and joins Carer Two on the other side of the bed.

- Carer Two flexes the Person's near knee.

- Both carers firmly grasp the low friction roller, establishing a good base of support with their feet or with a knee on the bed, and on 'Ready, Steady, Turn', both Carers step back while simultaneously pulling the roller slightly upwards. This backward and slightly upwards motion slides the Person while simultaneously turning him onto his side (Fig. 8.16).

- Remove the low friction roller(s) according to the manufacturer's instructions.

- Place pillows behind the Person and between his knees for support and roll the Person back onto the pillows at a 30 degree tilt (best practice to help reduce the risk of pressure sores). Do not position the pillows near his sacrum or any other bony prominence.

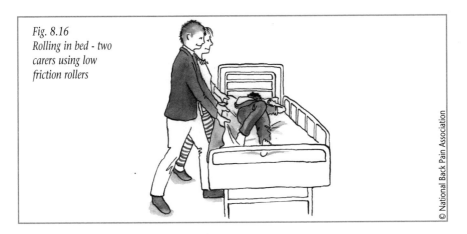

Fig. 8.16
Rolling in bed - two carers using low friction rollers

© National Back Pain Association

3.2.e. Mechanical roller and specialised beds (see Chapter 6: Equipment)

3.3. SITTING UP IN BED WITHOUT ASSISTANCE

3.3.a. Verbal Prompting

Using verbal prompting, a carer can encourage a Person to sit up in bed by rolling onto his side and pushing himself up. This requires less effort than trying to encourage a Person to sit forwards from a lying down position. Once he is in a sitting position, he can move back on his bottom. The Person can support himself when sitting by placing his hands on the bed just behind his hips. A rope ladder, bed lever or bed rails may help.

3.3.b. Rope ladder

The use of a rope ladder fixed to the bottom of the bed (Fig. 8.17) may allow the Person to pull himself forwards. The Person 'walks' his hands up the ladder by pulling with each hand in turn.

3.3.c. Bed lever or grab rail

Bed levers and grab rails firmly fixed in place allow the Person to obtain a firm grip on a secure object and pull himself up (Fig. 8.18).

3.3.d. Profiling beds, mattress inclinators and pillow lifters

The use of these items will reduce the need for the carer to manually assist the Person to sit forward, as the Person pushes buttons to operate and adjust the tilt of the bed, mattress and pillows.

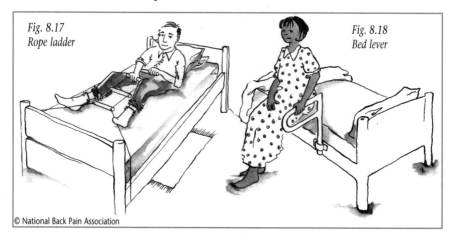

Fig. 8.17
Rope ladder

Fig. 8.18
Bed lever

3.4. SITTING UP IN BED WITH ASSISTANCE

3.4.a. Two carers

♦ As an interim procedure in the absence of mechanical device, place a soft handling sling behind the Person's scapulae (shoulder blades). This may be done by rolling the Person (see 3.2.a.). The sling must be held taut to avoid it slipping; ideally use a non-slip sling.

♦ The carers stand on opposite sides of the bed and face the head of the bed.

♦ Adjust the bed height to suit the shorter carer and to allow each carer's supporting foot to be flat on the floor. They kneel on the bed on their nearside leg, with their knee at the Person's hip/waist level.

♦ Both carers rise up off their heel with their spines in a naturally upright position, thus creating a space between the heel and buttocks.

♦ For comfort, the Person slightly bends one knee.

♦ Holding the soft handling sling with the near hand, the carers ensure the sling is taut and ask the Person to put his chin onto his chest.

♦ One carer says clearly 'Ready, Steady, Sit'.

♦ On the word 'Sit', both carers simultaneously transfer their body weight by sitting back onto their heels.

♦ The end result is both carers sitting down and the Person sitting up.

3.4.b. One carer

For this to be carried out safely, the Person must be in a half lying (or reclining) position and be able to provide the majority of effort; the carer the least amount. This should be determined after an in-depth assessment.

♦ The carer positions herself as in 3.4.a. above with both hands holding a soft handling sling.

♦ As the carer sits back her body weight is used to provide the minimal assistance needed to assist the Person to sit forward.

♦ If no handling sling is available, consider the use of a pillow as a last resort.

CAUTION: Do not use the manual techniques described above (3.4), if the Person resists forward movements.

3.5. MOVING UP IN BED

3.5.a Preventing slipping down the bed

1. Profiling beds

The use of these beds greatly reduces the risk of injury to the carer because she needs to do less moving and handling. At the same time, individual independence is increased for many people using them. Essentially, such beds have the capability of converting from a flat-bedded platform into a combination of positions. Profiling bed platforms come in either two, three or four sections. The choice of the platform positions can help prevent a Person slipping down in the bed or decrease the number of times they need to be repositioned. With the back rest up there is a tendency for the Person to slip down; raising the knee or foot section slightly will help reduce this.

N.B. DO NOT TILT the bed into a head down position to prevent slipping, as this may increase the blood pressure in a Person who is lying down and may lead to medical problems for some people[†].

2. One-way glide

This is an anti-slip low friction roller with velcro strips inside to allow single direction movement only. It will allow a Person to slide up but not slip down. CAUTION, use of a one-way glide may increase shearing* forces on the skin for some people and may not be recommended for people with fragile skin or poor circulation to the skin.

3. Careful positioning and choice of clothing

If a Person is initially correctly positioned either in bed or in a chair, the choice and positioning of clothing will help decrease the number of times the carer needs to reposition him. For example, if you use sufficient pillows when positioning a Person sitting up in bed they will give enough support to reduce slipping. Slipping will also be reduced if the person wears comfortable cotton clothing rather than slippery fabrics such as nylon.

3.5.b. Independent moving up the bed

1. Breaking down the move

It is often useful to break down a simple move such as this so that clear instructions can be provided to the Person. The Person will need reasonable upper limb strength and sitting balance to perform this move.

† *Pending EC bed manufacturers' change of standard to comply with Provision and Use of Work Equipment Regulations, 1992*
* *see Glossary*

- The Person leans forward in bed.

- The Person bends one or both knees and digs his heels into the bed.

- The Person places closed fists on the bed just behind his hips.

- By simultaneously pushing into the bed with the heels and down into the bed with the closed fists, the Person can lever himself back up the bed.

2. Rocking and shuffling his bottom

Just as it sounds, in this move the Person rocks onto one buttock while simultaneously moving the opposite buttock up the bed, then, maintaining momentum, rocks to the other side while simultaneously moving the opposite buttock up the bed and so on. This is repeated until the Person is in the desired position.

3.5.c Independent moving up the bed using handling aids

1. Using hand blocks

The move is the same as 3.5.b.2 above but the Person uses hand blocks instead of the closed fist. Hand blocks provide a higher lift of the Person's buttocks and make pushing down into the bed easier, by providing a stable base. These are particularly useful on soft mattresses.

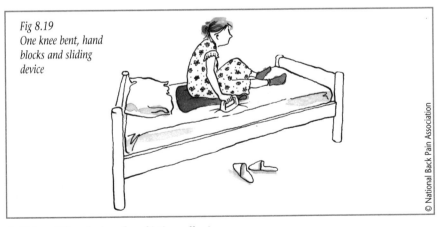

Fig 8.19
One knee bent, hand blocks and sliding device

© National Back Pain Association

2. Using sliding devices (low friction rollers)

You can place a sliding device under the Person's buttocks to assist the movement backwards. If the Person cannot bend one or both legs to help in the move, then a sliding device must be placed under the limb to prevent dragging of the heels on the bed. Hand blocks may also be useful in combination with sliding devices (Fig. 8.19).

3. By sitting to the edge of the bed

Getting to the edge of the bed from a lying to sitting position is described in section 4.2.a. To get back up in the bed the Person can:

♦ stand up, walk further up the bed and sit back down

♦ or shuffle up the bed

♦ or use a small sliding device under his buttocks and slide further up the bed. N.B. If using a sliding device, it must not hang over the bedside. Ensure the Person has adequate trunk control to prevent slipping off the bed.

3.5.d. Moving up the bed using a hoist

If the Person is unable to contribute significantly towards movement back up the bed, and if assisted techniques are difficult, then use a hoist. See Chapter 6: Equipment for in-depth explanation of hoists.

3.5.e. Move up the bed with assistance

1. Backward slide up the bed - seated Person with two carers (Figs. 8.21, 8.22, 8.23 and 8.24)

The use of a sitting slide technique to move a Person back up the bed will only be appropriate for a Person who is able to maintain a reasonable sitting balance.

♦ The carer places a sliding device under the Person as in 3.2.d, or the Person bridges (i.e. bends knees and raises his hips up off the bed, or is asked to lean side to side raising his buttocks) and the carer positions the sliding device underneath. It forms a loop along the length of the bed.

♦ A sliding device must also be placed under the Person's legs and heels if he is unable to help by digging his heels into the bed during the manoeuvre. The position of the sliding device is important. Some sliding devices indicate the position where the Person's hips should rest. For those that do not, it is easiest to position the device where it is intended that the Person should be at the end of the move. It can then be rolled back down under the Person's hips and removed after the Person has been repositioned.

♦ If necessary, the Person is then brought to a sitting position as in 3.4.a.

♦ Both carers now turn and face the bottom of the bed and position their near knee and lower leg on the bed just behind the Person's hips, ensuring their knees are under the sliding device not on top of it. The other foot is placed firmly on the floor.

♦ The carers hold the handles of the sliding device with their near hands. If there are no handles, the carer at the hip level rolls the top layer only of the sliding device and grasps it firmly (Fig. 8.20).

♦ The carers may gently: hold the Person's shoulder (Figs. 8.23 and 8.24), hold his hand or, if he feels stable, position his hands in his lap (Figs. 8.23 and 8.24) while the carers maintain their own natural curves of the spine in an upright posture.

♦ Once in position, the carers rise up off their heels, both carers holding the sliding device taut (Fig. 8.20).

♦ One carer says clearly 'Ready, Steady, Slide' and on the word 'Slide' both carers sit back simultaneously onto their heels, and the Person slides up the bed.

♦ More than one move up the bed may be needed. Take care not to overshoot as this may cause the carers to twist.

♦ Remove the sliding device following the manufacturer's instructions.

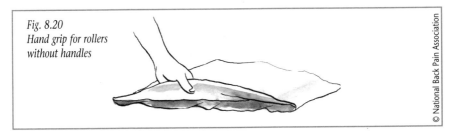

Fig. 8.20
Hand grip for rollers
without handles

© National Back Pain Association

CAUTION: With techniques which require two carers and/or when working with an obese Person, it is possible that the bed may tip as the carers sit back. Always check the weight limit of the bed.

2. Backward slide up the bed - seated Person with one carer

This technique should be used with caution as it relies on the Person usefully participating by using his legs to help push himself up the bed. The Person, therefore, needs to be able to understand the verbal instructions and commands used by the carer during the move.

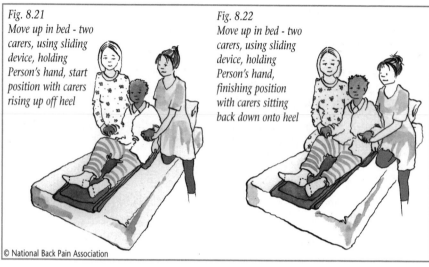

Fig. 8.21
Move up in bed - two carers, using sliding device, holding Person's hand, start position with carers rising up off heel

Fig. 8.22
Move up in bed - two carers, using sliding device, holding Person's hand, finishing position with carers sitting back down onto heel

© National Back Pain Association

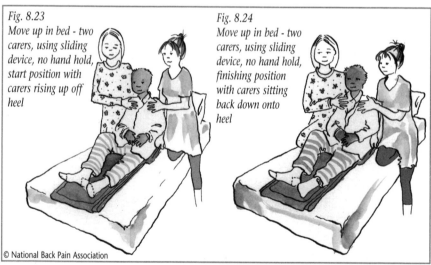

Fig. 8.23
Move up in bed - two carers, using sliding device, no hand hold, start position with carers rising up off heel

Fig. 8.24
Move up in bed - two carers, using sliding device, no hand hold, finishing position with carers sitting back down onto heel

© National Back Pain Association

♦ Position a sliding device under the Person's bottom as in 3.5.e.1 above.

♦ The carer positions herself just behind and to one side of the Person's hip.

♦ The carer places her near knee and lower leg on the bed while facing the foot of the bed, ensuring her knee is under the sliding device not on top of it. She places the other foot firmly on the floor.

♦ The carer sits up off her heel.

- The carer holds each side of the sliding device with her hands.

- Once in position, the carer rises up off of her heel and holds the sliding device tautly in position.

- The carer says clearly 'Ready, Steady, Slide' and, on the word 'Slide', she sits back onto her heel as the Person simultaneously pushes up the bed by digging his heels into the mattress.

- More than one move up the bed may be needed. Take care not to overshoot and twist.

- Remove the sliding device by following the manufacturer's instructions.

3. Supine slide (Person lying down) with two carers -using a sliding device (Fig. 8.25)

Ideally, place two sliding sheets with handles underneath the Person in bed. Do this by turning the Person as noted in 3.1.c. above. If necessary, use one full-length low friction roller (one with the opening at the Person's sides), or a series of smaller sliding devices ensuring the Person's head, trunk, hips and heels are on a sliding device surface.

- Raise the bed to optimal working height for the carers and both carers position themselves on the same side of the bed in the direction of travel.

- Once the sliding devices are correctly positioned, the carers position themselves either side of the bed with their near knee at the Person's shoulder level and their far foot on the floor in front of them.

- With their near hands, the carers hold the handle at the Person's shoulder level (the carers' knee). If the device does not have handles they hold it directly.

- The carers then hold the handle with their far hands (or sliding device) next to the Person's hip. A pull strap attached to the handle would prevent any twisting or stretching by the carers, but this must be held taut and not wrapped around the carers' hands (Fig. 8.25).

♦ The carers must take care to avoid the Person's head hitting the headboard, by moving in small stages.

♦ The movement is provided by the carers simultaneously sitting back onto their heels.

♦ Remove the sliding devices as soon as the move is completed.

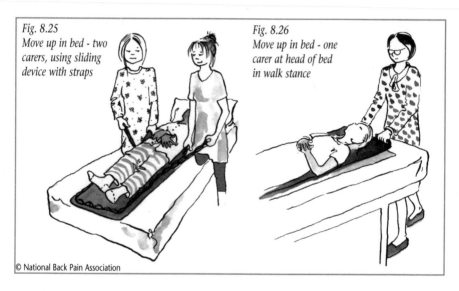

Fig. 8.25
Move up in bed - two carers, using sliding device with straps

Fig. 8.26
Move up in bed - one carer at head of bed in walk stance

© National Back Pain Association

The same technique can be modified by having carers in a walk stance by the side of the bed, or standing at the head of the bed and pulling the Person towards them using the handles; the slide is achieved by using the attached pull straps on the top sliding device. A single carer can perform this manoeuvre if the Person is small (within her individual capabilities) and there is good access at the head of the bed (Fig. 8.26).

If the Person is difficult to move, then a hoist will be required. If sitting is inappropriate and there is a need to maintain a supine (lying down) position, then a stretcher attachment may need to be used.

4. Moving down the bed with assistance - two carers using sliding devices

The reverse of 3. above is performed.

3.6. UNSAFE TECHNIQUES (See also section 11)

- ⊘ UNSAFE TECHNIQUE - AUSTRALIAN/ SHOULDER LIFT or AUSTRALIAN / SHOULDER SLIDE
- ⊘ UNSAFE TECHNIQUE - UNDERARM DRAG LIFT
- ⊘ UNSAFE TECHNIQUE - ORTHODOX / CRADLE LIFT
- ⊘ UNSAFE TECHNIQUE - USING LINEN SHEETS TO LIFT OR DRAG

4 Sitting to the edge of the bed

4.1. SITTING TO THE EDGE OF THE BED WITHOUT ASSISTANCE

The Person requires upper limb strength and good sitting balance.

4.1.a. Side lying position

Described for a Person getting out of bed onto their left side.

- ♦ With his knees bent, the Person should roll onto his left side and push his feet near to the edge of the bed.

- ♦ The Person places his right arm across his body and positions his right hand on the mattress at shoulder level ready to use it to push.

- ♦ The Person simultaneously drops his legs over the side of the bed and, using his right hand, pushes himself sideways and upwards into a sitting position using his left elbow as a lever (Figs. 8.27 and 8.28).

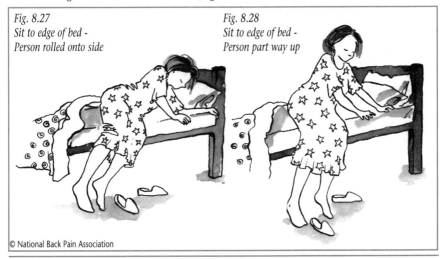

Fig. 8.27
Sit to edge of bed -
Person rolled onto side

Fig. 8.28
Sit to edge of bed -
Person part way up

4.2. SITTING TO THE EDGE OF THE BED WITH ASSISTANCE

The Person requires upper limb strength and good sitting balance.

4.2.a. Side lying position with one carer assisting

Described for a Person getting out of bed onto their left side. If the bed is height-adjustable, then adjust it to allow the carer to provide some assistance without needing to stoop or twist.

♦ With his knees bent, the Person rolls onto his left side and pushes his feet near to the edge of the bed.

♦ The Person places his right arm across his body and positions his hand on the mattress near to the level of his chest and shoulder.

♦ The Person simultaneously drops his legs over the side of the bed and, using his right hand, pushes himself sideways and upwards into a sitting position using the left elbow as a lever, while the carer simultaneously pushes up on the Person's left shoulder (Fig. 8.29a).

♦ The carer assists by holding both the Person's shoulders (Fig. 8.29b).

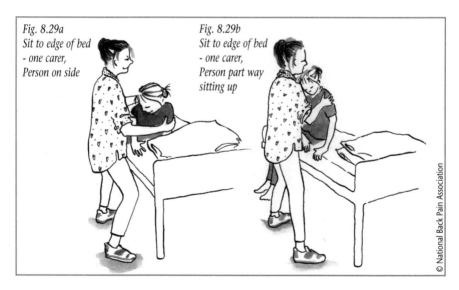

Fig. 8.29a
Sit to edge of bed
- one carer,
Person on side

Fig. 8.29b
Sit to edge of bed
- one carer,
Person part way
sitting up

© National Back Pain Association

The movement must be well co-ordinated. The carer must adopt a wide and stable base of foot support and be able to transfer her weight from side to side in the process. A second carer may need to assist taking the legs off of the bed as the

Person sits up. If the carer places a soft handling sling under the calves, it will help reduce the need to stoop (see 4.2.b.).

CAUTION: On no account should the carer lift the whole or the bulk of the Person's weight from a lying to a sitting position. If more assistance is required then use a mechanical aid such as a mattress inclinator (See Chapter 6: Equipment).

4.2.b. Assisting to sit to the edge of the bed with turning disc or sliding device (Fig. 8.30)

1.   The Person requires upper limb strength and good sitting balance. As above (3.5.e.1), position a turning disc or sliding device under the Person's buttocks to facilitate a swivel motion to bring him to a sitting position on the edge of the bed. You can also place a sliding device underneath the feet to facilitate movement of the legs to and from the edge of the bed.

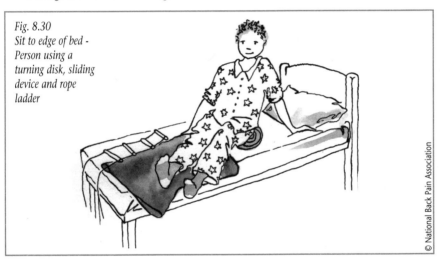

Fig. 8.30
Sit to edge of bed -
Person using a
turning disk, sliding
device and rope
ladder

© National Back Pain Association

2.   If the Person has sitting balance but is unable to move his legs off the bed, position a low friction roller under his bottom and a soft handling sling under his calves (Fig. 8.31). Maintaining her back in a normal upright position, the carer lifts the handling sling while simultaneously turning the Person to the side of the bed. Once the Person's legs are over the side, the carer maintains her back in a normal upright position and bends her knees while lowering the handling sling under the Person's calves (Fig. 8.32).

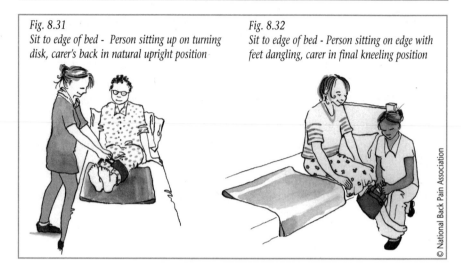

Fig. 8.31
Sit to edge of bed - Person sitting up on turning disk, carer's back in natural upright position

Fig. 8.32
Sit to edge of bed - Person sitting on edge with feet dangling, carer in final kneeling position

© National Back Pain Association

3.   If the Person has sitting and standing balance but is unable to move his legs back onto the bed, then you must consider a mechanical system (e.g. powered leg lifters (see Chapter 6: Equipment)). However, if you cannot avoid lifting the legs, then use a reverse procedure as described in 4.2.b.2 above.

5. Transfers

For example, bed to commode, wheelchair to bed, wheelchair to sofa.

5.1. WEIGHTBEARING TRANSFERS WITHOUT ASSISTANCE

5.1.a. Independent (may need verbal prompting or encouragement)

With verbal prompting, a Person may be able to transfer independently.

♦   Firstly, consider the position of chairs, wheelchairs, chair raisers.

♦   See 1.2. above.

♦   Once standing, the Person can step round to the chair/commode/etc. This will be made easier if the distance to walk is as short as possible.

5.1.b. Independent with aids

If the Person is unable to step round once standing, then consider the use of aids e.g. turning plate, bridging boards. You can place a turning plate (turntable) under the feet close to the destination (chair/toilet/etc.). You can also use a bridging board (Fig 8.33) (see 5.3.b and Fig. 8.35 for explanation).

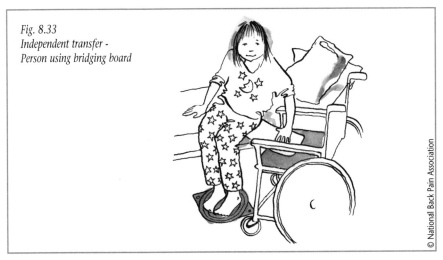

Fig. 8.33
Independent transfer -
Person using bridging board

© National Back Pain Association

5.2. WEIGHTBEARING TRANSFERS WITH ASSISTANCE - CHAIR TO CHAIR

5.2.a. Transfers aids

Several transfer aids are available to assist standing and transferring a Person. The following are described in more detail in the techniques below:

♦ standing hoists

♦ mobile standing prop.

5.2.b. Two carers with a Person able to walk

♦ Position furniture so that both carers can get to each side of the chair, while keeping the distance to be moved to a minimum.

♦ The use of a handling belt is preferred.

♦ Use the technique described in 1.4.b. above to bring the Person to a standing position.

♦ Pause to allow the Person to get his balance.

♦ Both carers and the Person walk round together using an appropriate handhold, holding onto walking aids if necessary. If this is a move to the commode or toilet, then you will will need to consider clothing adjustment (see Toileting: Section 9 below).

5.2.c. One carer with a Person able to walk

♦ One carer should do this only if the Person is able to fully weightbear and move with minimal assistance.

♦ Use a handling belt if not contraindicated.

♦ Position furniture to allow the carer access to the side of the chair.

♦ Position the destination chair/commode/etc. close by.

♦ Use the technique described in 1.4.b above to bring the Person to a standing position and walk him round to chair/commode/etc.

♦ The carer must be able to stay at the Person's side when he sits down unless he can let go and hold onto the arm of the chair to lower himself. The carer must maintain good posture as the Person sits down.

♦ Reverse the procedure of 1.4.b. above to assist the Person to sit down.

5.2.d.. Two carers assisting a Person up from a bed with a Person able to walk (Figs. 8.34a and 8.34b)

♦ Use a handling belt if not contraindicated.

♦ Position the destination chair/commode/etc. close by with enough room for a carer to stay at each side of the Person during the transfer.

♦ Both carers sit on the bed, one on either side of the Person.

♦ The carers hold the handling belt with the near hand and the Person's hand with their other hand. Alternatively they can encourage the Person to push up by placing his hands on his thighs. A rocking action may help.

♦ Once standing, pause to allow the Person to get his balance, and then walk him round to the chair/commode/etc.

♦ The carers must be able to stay at the Person's side when he sits down unless he can let go and hold onto the arm of the chair and lower himself. Carers must maintain good posture as the Person sits down.

♦ Reverse the procedure of 1.4.b. above to assist the Person to sit down.

N.B. If one carer is performing this transfer technique, the Person must be able to fully weightbear and move with minimal assistance. The carer should sit on the bed and, if the Person has one weaker side, the carer should sit at that weak side.

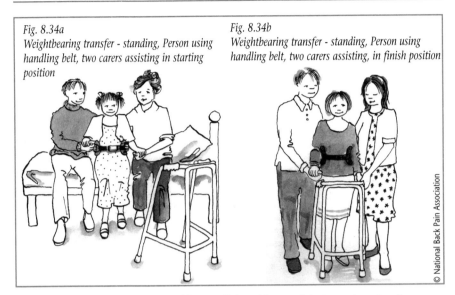

Fig. 8.34a
Weightbearing transfer - standing, Person using handling belt, two carers assisting in starting position

Fig. 8.34b
Weightbearing transfer - standing, Person using handling belt, two carers assisting, in finish position

© National Back Pain Association

5.2.e. Two carers with a Person unable to walk but able to weight bear when standing

1. Wheeled appliance

- The Person must be able to weightbear.

- Use the technique described in 1.3.b above to bring the Person to a standing position.

- Move the wheeled appliance (e.g. commode) in behind the Person (this may require 3 carers).

- Reverse the procedure of 1.3.b above to assist the Person to sit down (Figs. 8.7 - 8.10).

2. Turning plate

This must be used with caution. A second carer should be available to position the destination chair directly behind and touching the Person.

- Position the destination chair/commode/etc. close by leaving enough room for a carer to stay at each side of the Person during the transfer.

- Position a large turning plate under the Person's feet.

- Carer Two places one foot on the turning plate to prevent it from turning while the person is standing up. Once the person is standing, Carer Two removes her foot.

- Use the technique described in 1.3. above to bring the Person to a standing position (Fig. 8.7).

- Carer One positions one hand on the front of the Person's hip and her other hand on the back of the opposite hip and pulls/pushes his hips in the direction of travel.

- Reverse the procedure of 1.3.b. above to assist the Person to sit down.

5.3. NON-WEIGHTBEARING TRANSFERS WITHOUT ASSISTANCE

5.3.a. Independent non-weightbearing transfer

- A Person with good upper body strength may be able to shuffle sideways from one surface to another independently. This could be done with or without a sliding board and is extremely useful for a Person who has had a limb amputated.

- A turning plate under the Person's foot or feet may ease the movement.

- A carer or carers may assist with a handling belt.

5.3.b. One carer with a Person unable to walk or stand but with good upper body strength

- Use a bridging board and handling belt if not contraindicated.

- The Person must have good sitting balance, good upper body strength, understand simple instructions and be able to usefully participate in the move.

- Position the destination chair/commode/etc. close by with one end of the bridging board securely under the Person's buttock nearest to the transfer surface.

- Position the other end of the bridging board securely on the chair/ commode/ toilet/ etc. so that it bridges the gap (to prevent movement of the board when the receiving surface is uneven e.g. a toilet seat, a non-slip netting can be rolled up under the board).

- A turning plate positioned under the Person's feet may be useful to assist movement (Fig. 8.35).

- The carer stands in the gap behind the Person and between the two surfaces, then assists the Person across the board by holding onto the handling belt (moving with the Person to reach the destination chair). The carer must ensure she transfers her weight and does not twist her spine.

- If the move is more than one carer can do, use a hoist.

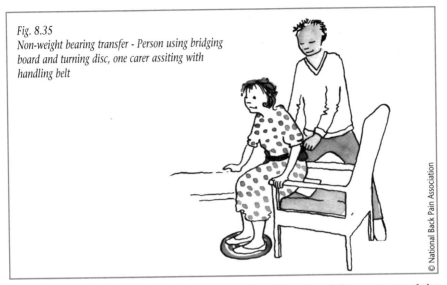

Fig. 8.35
Non-weight bearing transfer - Person using bridging board and turning disc, one carer assiting with handling belt

© National Back Pain Association

As with all techniques, for safety the carer should make a full assessment of the Person prior to using this technique to be sure that only one carer is required.

5.3.c. Mechanical Assistance

Hoists may be used for non-weightbearing transfers (see Chapter 6: Equipment).

5.4 UNSAFE TECHNIQUES (See also Section 11)

- ✪ UNSAFE TECHNIQUE - AUSTRALIAN / SHOULDER LIFT

- ✪ UNSAFE TECHNIQUE - UNDERARM DRAG

- ✪ UNSAFE TECHNIQUE - PIVOT TRANSFER / STANDING TRANSFER / BEAR HUG

- ✪ UNSAFE TECHNIQUE - ARM AND LEG LUG

6. A falling or fallen Person

There are several techniques in current practice and each one recognises that trying to stop a falling Person is very unsafe and likely to lead to injury to the carer and possibly to the Person himself. It is impossible to set out parameters dealing with all situations and the ones listed below are set in a practical environment and do not deal with life-threatening situations. The following is intended as a guide only and is by no means exhaustive. The techniques described should only be used after specific training and completing a moving and handling assessment for the Person.

6.1. ASSESSMENT

Areas to be covered by assessment to establish the risk of falling include:

- previous history of falling

- cognitive* understanding - what is the Person's level of understanding of what is expected of him and how much is he able to co-operate

- physical and mental co-ordination (i.e. alert and not confused)

- weightbearing abilities including balance, strength, medical condition and spasticity (or sudden muscle movement)

- walking aids used including walking frames, walking sticks, callipers, slippery footwear, prosthesis, etc.

- environmental hazards such as loose carpets or rugs, electric fires or sharp objects, clothing, pets underfoot

- carer's capabilities including clothing and footwear.

6.2. TECHNIQUES

6.2.a. Falling Person - out of the carer's reach

It is unrealistic to physically assist the Person - there is not enough time to reach him and too great a distance to reach and stretch. If there is no immediate danger of the Person striking a fixed or immovable object, allow him to fall.

6.2.b. Falling Person - carer within close proximity but not physically touching or assisting at the time of the fall

The carer may be able to do one of the following:

- think ahead and where possible, remove dangerous objects within the environment prior to the Person walking in the area

- redirect the fall by pushing or pulling the Person away from dangerous or immovable objects.

6.2.c. Falling Person - carer is in physical contact or delivering care at the time of the fall

There is no one safe way of dealing with the falling Person even if the carer is in close physical contact at the time. The following guidelines maybe helpful (Figs. 8.36 and 8.37).

- The carer may have more control if she positions herself behind the falling Person rather than in front.

- The carer has both hands open while taking a step backwards but keeping close to the Person.

- The carer is likely to have more control holding the Person's torso rather than his arms.

- The carer bends her knees and maintains a stable base to help protect her back while allowing the Person to slide to the floor.

- The carer supports the Person's head where possible.

- The carer allows the Person to fall rather than supporting them in an upright or slumped position.

- Do not take all of the Person's weight.

- When the Person is sitting on the floor and leaning against the carer, the carer may then step back and kneel down while protecting the Person's head and maintaining her normal back position (Fig. 8.38).

- Then follow recommendations in 7. below.

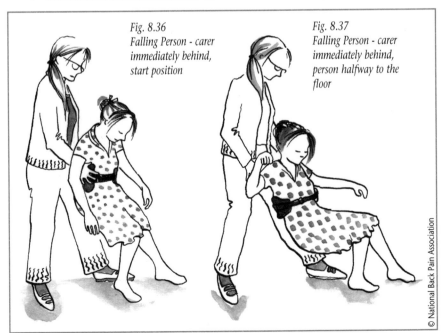

Fig. 8.36
Falling Person - carer immediately behind, start position

Fig. 8.37
Falling Person - carer immediately behind, person halfway to the floor

© National Back Pain Association

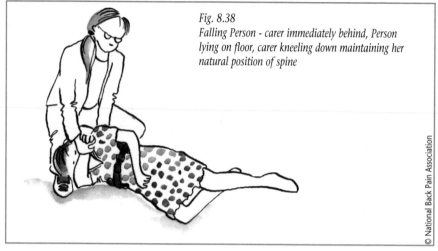

Fig. 8.38
Falling Person - carer immediately behind, Person lying on floor, carer kneeling down maintaining her natural position of spine

© National Back Pain Association

6.3 UNSAFE TECHNIQUES (See Section 11)

    ✪ UNSAFE TECHNIQUE - CATCHING THE FALLING PERSON

    ✪ UNSAFE TECHNIQUE - TRYING TO HOLD A COLLAPSED PERSON UPRIGHT

7. Assisting the fallen Person up from the floor

7.1. BEING AWARE

Carers who work with People who walk or do standing transfers must always be aware of the possibility of a fall. Managers must ensure that there is a safe strategy in place to enable carers to cope with a Person at high risk of falling. People receiving care should also be aware of such strategies so that they do not put pressure on carers to inappropriately assist or lift them up from the floor. Unless the fallen Person is in immediate and further danger, then there is no need to hurry to get him up off the floor. He cannot fall any further and acting without careful assessment could cause injury to both him and the carer.

7.1.a. Assessment

If you come across a Person on the floor or ground and did not witness the event which brought him to the ground, then first ensure there are no dangers in approaching him (e.g. are there live electrical leads touching him). Make the area safe first and check that no further danger exists. Call for assistance. A medical and physical assessment of the fallen Person should be undertaken immediately. If the

Person is unconscious, the priority is to follow the recommended procedures for First Aid and place him in the Recovery Position. First Aid is beyond the remit of this book and you should seek advice and training on this issue from your manager. When in doubt, or if you are worried about the medical status of the Person, then call 999. Do not attempt to lift or move the Person without the appropriate equipment and before sufficient help has arrived unless there are overriding factors (fire/smoke, imminent collapse of the building, flooding/drowning, bombs/explosions, etc.).

7.2. THE UNINJURED CONSCIOUS FALLEN PERSON

7.2.a. Independent transfer

This technique is useful to teach to People who live alone and who regularly fall. It provides reassurance to them that they can get up by themselves and do not always have to wait for help to arrive.

- Stay calm and remain with the Person, don't let him hurry to get up.

- Place a pillow under the Person's head and wait until he feels ready to try to get up.

- Encourage the Person to bend up both knees (one at a time) and roll onto his side, and then push up into a side sitting position.

- When ready, ask him to roll onto all fours.

- Bring a low stable chair or stool to the Person's side.

- Encourage the Person to place his near hand on the seat and bring his near leg through so that he is able push up onto the near foot.

- Ask the Person to push down on his raised knee with his other hand.

- Encourage the Person to push down on the seat and through his foot while swinging his hips round to sit onto the seat (Figs. 8.39, 8.40 and 8.41).

A carer should never manually lift a fallen Person up from the floor except in a life-threatening emergency, and then only after thorough assessment.

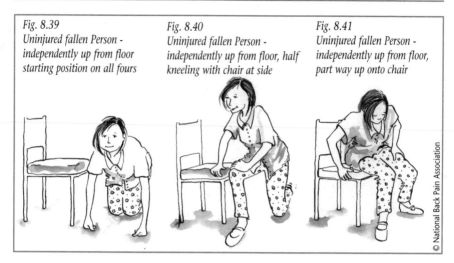

Fig. 8.39
Uninjured fallen Person -
independently up from floor
starting position on all fours

Fig. 8.40
Uninjured fallen Person -
independently up from floor, half
kneeling with chair at side

Fig. 8.41
Uninjured fallen Person -
independently up from floor,
part way up onto chair

© National Back Pain Association

7.3. EMERGENCY LIFTING CUSHIONS / POWERED AIR RAISING DEVICES (See Chapter 5)

If the fallen Person has sitting balance and trunk control and can stabilise himself using his arms, then a powered air raising device can be used (Fig. 8.42). This has the benefit of being reasonably portable and can enable a Person to get on or off the floor following a fall. Such devices often work on rechargeable power units so they can be used anywhere. An example for the use of this device is for a wheelchair-dependent Person who wishes to play with his children on the ground outdoors. In order to ensure stability, there needs to be some assistance from a second person when using the air raising device (see Chapter 6: Equipment).

There are emergency air raising devices available for People who need back support (i.e. who lean back but have no sitting balance and do not fall to the left or right). Refer to a Disabled Living Foundation Centre for more information.

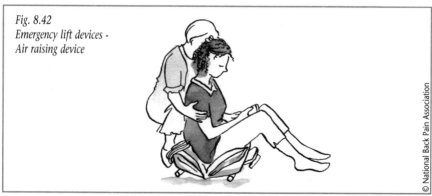

Fig. 8.42
Emergency lift devices -
Air raising device

© National Back Pain Association

7.4. RESTRICTED ACCESS TO A FALLEN PERSON

See Special Situations, Section 10 below.

7.5. ASSISTED TRANSFERS FROM THE FLOOR

7.5.a. Hoist (sling or stretcher)

A hoist provides a safe method of mechanically lifting a Person up from the floor. In most cases a fabric sling is sufficient, however, following a cardiac arrest (heart attack), a stretcher sling will be needed. Access slings that have little support should not be used to raise People from the floor. In a cardiac arrest situation in the community, call the ambulance service on 999 and do not attempt to move the Person even following successful resuscitation.

N.B. Different makes of hoist use different approaches to moving a Person off the floor and different requirements on applying the brakes or not. Some use an approach from the direction of the Person's feet, some from the head or sideways with the Person's knees raised for one of the hoist legs to fit under them. Others recommend either approach depending on the circumstances. You should determine the manufacturer's recommendations and practise following these before encountering a real situation.

7.5.b. Transfers using a fabric sling with the hoist (Figs. 8.43a and 8.43b)

Position the fabric sling in one of two ways. Either roll the Person onto it or ask him to sit forwards, position the sling and then support him in a sitting position using a bean bag or the back of an upturned chair. If necessary, the carer can fully kneel with the Person's head and shoulders resting on their knees. This provides reassurance for the fallen Person and can also make it easier to connect the sling to the hoist at the shoulders. The carer must avoid lifting the head and shoulders while in a kneeling position. Wait for assistance.

Once the Person is hoisted into a chair, it may be necessary to readjust the loops to achieve an upright posture for sitting in the chair.

Always follow the manufacturers' instructions on the use of hoists and slings. These should be accessible to carers to read.

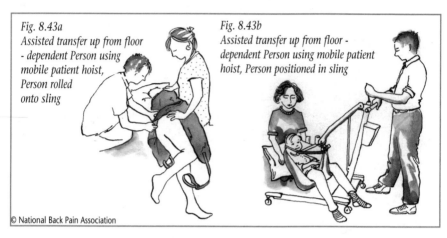

Fig. 8.43a
Assisted transfer up from floor
- dependent Person using
mobile patient hoist,
Person rolled
onto sling

Fig. 8.43b
Assisted transfer up from floor -
dependent Person using mobile patient
hoist, Person positioned in sling

© National Back Pain Association

7.6 UNSAFE TECHNIQUES (See also Section 11)

- ✪ UNSAFE TECHNIQUE - ARM AND LEG LUG

- ✪ UNSAFE TECHNIQUE - UNDERARM DRAG LIFT

- ✪ UNSAFE TECHNIQUE - ONE, TWO, THREE, FOUR OR MORE PHYSICALLY LIFT

- ✪ UNSAFE TECHNIQUE - SHOULDER LIFT

- ✪ UNSAFE TECHNIQUE - CANVAS AND POLES

8. Repositioning in a chair

If People slump too much in a chair, there is a danger that they can slip to the floor. A lack of sitting balance or trunk control can cause this. It may be that the Person's clothing is slippery or shiny, or he is simply slipping on the seating surface. It is sometimes difficult to position people to the back of their chair correctly when using a hoist and the sling is frequently removed before discovering the Person is not positioned correctly. Carers must not be tempted to manually lift the Person back once the sling has been removed. There are several ways to reposition or position a Person so that he is sitting right at the back of the chair.

8.1. PREVENTING THE SLIP (Fig. 8.44)

♦ Avoid slippery coverings on seats.

♦ Avoid surfaces that slope downwards to the front of the chair, especially when the Person is wearing clothing made of a slippery fabric.

♦ Ensure the seat is the right size, shape and depth for the Person and that he can sit supported with his feet on the floor or on a footstool or on the footplate/footrest).

♦ A One-Way glide can be used to help prevent slipping. Some of these glides are padded with sheepskin or gel packs to provide some protection against constant pressure. Some One-way glides are available with handles. To reposition a One-way glide without handles, the carer kneels down in front of the Person and applies pressure through the Person's knees to slide him back in the chair. One-way glides can also be useful to achieve a good seated position when hoisting.

♦ Lean the Person forward prior to sliding him back in the chair.

♦ Take care not to lift the Person but to slide them.

♦ Do not put a One-way glide on top of pressure relieving seating.

CAUTION, use of a One-way glide may not be recommended for people with fragile skin or poor circulation to the skin.

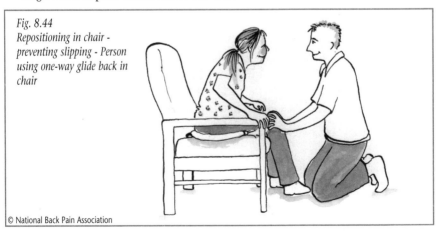

Fig. 8.44
Repositioning in chair - preventing slipping - Person using one-way glide back in chair

It is important to avoid the Underarm Drag Lift, Top and Tail Lift or the Arm and Leg Lug to lift and reposition People.

8.1.a. Repeated slipping

If there is repeated slipping even after following the steps above, it may be necessary to have a chair that tilts back completely, or have a wedge on the seat to raise the front of the chair seat. If a wedge is used, be careful of pressure areas as the wedge shifts the weight of the Person concentrating it more under his buttocks.

8.2. REPOSITIONING WITHOUT ASSISTANCE

8.2.a. Verbal encouragement

◆ Encourage the Person to bend both knees so that his feet are on the floor (as for sitting to standing).

◆ Encourage him to lean forwards and then either:

   ◆ stand up and sit down again with his buttocks as far back in the chair as possible

   ◆ shuffle his buttocks back in the chair

◆ Alternatively, the chair can be brought closer to the Person if he is unable to step back.

◆ If required, you can assist him when he is standing as described in 1.3.6. above.

8.3. REPOSITIONING USING HANDLING AIDS (See Chapter 5)

8.3.a. Standing hoist or sling hoist

If using a sling hoist for repositioning a Person in a wheelchair with a tilt bar, then the chair can be tilted backwards as he is being lowered into the wheelchair. This will facilitate positioning into the back of the wheelchair. (N.B. This should not be used when repositioning a Person in a large armchair.)

8.3.b. Low friction roller or sliding device

This technique is for a Person able to co-operate and requires a minimum of two carers. One carer must always remain in a kneeling position in front of the seated Person to prevent him slipping further forwards onto the slide. If necessary, place a pillow in front of the Person's knees for comfort when pushing.

◆ Roll the sliding device in half.

◆ Encourage the Person to shuffle or lean from side to side while inserting the sliding device underneath his buttocks from either side, ensuring it is positioned in the correct manner with the open sides to the sides of the chair.

♦ The majority of the sliding device should be behind the Person on the seat.

♦ Once in place, ask the Person to lean forwards and either have him push himself back or, so long as the Person does not have painful knees or hips, apply gentle pressure through his thighs/knees towards the back of the chair (Fig. 8.45).

♦ If a third person is present then two carers each positioned on opposite sides can pull on the side of the sliding device (or on the handles if available) and slide the Person back in the chair. While pulling the sliding device both carers must adopt a walk stance and use their body weight to assist.

♦ Take care to slide the Person, not to lift him.

♦ A carer must always remain kneeling in front of the Person until the sliding device is removed.

♦ Never lean over a high backed chair to pull a Person back in a chair even with a sliding device.

♦ To remove the sliding device, pull on the underneath layer of material and draw out from under the Person towards the back of the chair.

Fig. 8.45
Repositioning in chair - Person on sliding device , carer pushing on knees

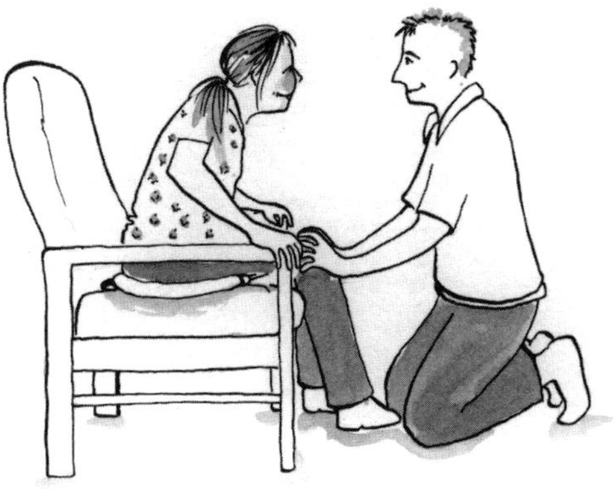

© National Back Pain Association

8.4. REPOSITIONING WITH ASSISTANCE WITHOUT HANDLING AIDS

For unusual circumstances when the techniques above are inappropriate or equipment is not available, it may be possible to assist a Person to 'bottom walk' or 'hip hitch' back into the chair.

♦ The carer should be in front of the Person in a high kneeling position (i.e. kneeling up, not sitting on her heels).

♦ The Person is asked to lean to one side and 'walk' or 'hip hitch' the opposite buttock backwards. The carer's role is to guide this manoeuvre towards the back of the chair by either facilitating at the Person's buttock or by gentle pressure through his knee towards the back of the chair.

♦ The Person then lifts the opposite buttock and leans to the other side; again the carer applies gentle pressure through his knee towards the back of the chair.

♦ The Person repeats the same manoeuvres on opposite hips/buttocks until he reaches the back of the chair.

8.5 UNSAFE TECHNIQUES (See also Section 11)

- ○ UNSAFE TECHNIQUE - PIVOT TRANSFER / BEAR HUG / STANDING TRANSFER

- ○ UNSAFE TECHNIQUE - UNDERARM DRAG

- ○ UNSAFE TECHNIQUE - MANUAL LIFTING OF ALL OR MOST OF PERSON'S FULL WEIGHT

- ○ UNSAFE TECHNIQUE - ARM AND LEG LUG

- ○ UNSAFE TECHNIQUE - TOP AND TAIL

9. Toileting

People often need help to use the toilet. It is useful to enlist the help of an occupational therapist who has a good working knowledge of useful equipment and adaptations in and around the toilet/bathroom area. An occupational therapist may consider some of the following:

♦ fixed or fold down grab rails

♦ toilet seat raisers of varying heights

♦ an automatic toilet that cleans and dries the Person while he is sitting on the toilet. (This helps preserve independence, privacy and dignity, and is welcomed by many people. It may not be as helpful for a Person who has sudden muscle spasms as the water jet may stimulate muscle spasm.)

♦ raiser toilet seats to assist the Person to stand afterwards

♦ bathroom or toilet adaptations including repositioning of furniture and appliances to provide better access for the Person and carer.

It is important that you make a detailed assessment before any equipment or adaptations are installed. All equipment or adaptations must be properly fitted and the Person must be taught how to use them. In many cases, with the right equipment or adaptations, people can independently transfer to and from the toilet.

9.1. ADAPTIVE CLOTHING (Fig. 8.46 a-e)

It is often difficult to adjust a Perons's clothing when using the toilet. To help, many People opt not to wear any undergarments and choose to wear a soft, loose garment like jogging trousers. Standard clothing can sometimes be adapted to facilitate use of the toilet. For example:

1.   For women, underwear is available with a drop down edge at the front of the reinforced gusset secured with a Velcro strip. The Velcro strip must be positioned with the hooks facing away from the Person so that the soft loop side can be secured by pressing into place against the Person. Trousers with a drop down edge are also available (Fig. 8.46a). This is useful if using a handle held urinal with a tube leading to a toilet pan. This involves no transferring of the Person.

2.   Pants or trousers can be split at the back to preserve dignity at the front but allow easier access from behind (Fig. 8.46b).

3.   An 'all-in-one' undergarment (teddy) with fastenings at the crotch or crotchless pants can provide easier access (Fig. 8.46c).

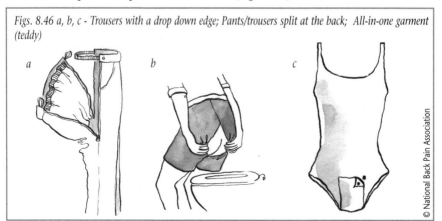

Figs. 8.46 a, b, c - Trousers with a drop down edge; Pants/trousers split at the back; All-in-one garment (teddy)

a   *b*   *c*

© National Back Pain Association

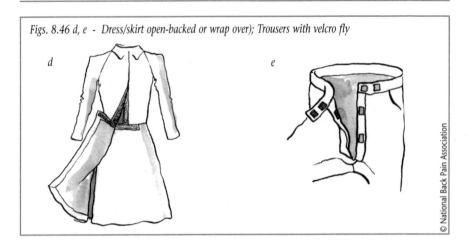

Figs. 8.46 d, e - Dress/skirt open-backed or wrap over); Trousers with velcro fly

d

e

© National Back Pain Association

4. Dresses or skirts can be open backed or wrap-over (Fig. 8.46d).

5. Zip flies for men can be replaced by Velcro that can provide quicker and easier access (Fig. 8.46e).

If standard undergarments are worn and the Person is unable to stand, it may be necessary to ask the Person to rock from side to side or lean over to one side at a time while a carer adjusts clothing at the opposite side. This needs to be done in stages; the carer should be careful to adopt a posture that does not involve stooping and twisting. It is often necessary to kneel down next to the Person to adjust clothing (Fig. 8.47).

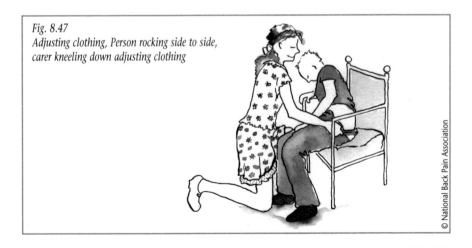

Fig. 8.47
Adjusting clothing, Person rocking side to side, carer kneeling down adjusting clothing

© National Back Pain Association

9.2. TRANSFERS ONTO THE TOILET WITH ASSISTANCE

For these transfers the techniques in 1.4. and 5.1. & 5.2. are used. Whichever method is chosen after an assessment of the capabilities and limitations of both the Person and carer(s), one important rule is NEVER PROVIDE SUPPORT TO A PERSON IN A STANDING POSITION WHILE PROVIDING PERSONAL HYGIENE CARE OR ADJUSTING CLOTHING AT THE SAME TIME. This inevitably places the carer in a twisting and stooping posture while she is off balance and trying to support a Person who at that moment is unstable. Following a detailed assessment, you can support a Person who can stand by the following methods:

♦ a standing hoist

♦ suitably placed grab rails (Fig. 8.48)

♦ walking aids (Fig. 8.49)

♦ rigid standing prop

♦ a second carer who does not assist with the personal hygiene or clothing adjustment. (A handling belt may be useful to assist the second carer by providing a more secure grip.)

If the Person can weightbear, all of these methods will enable full access for adjusting clothing or replacing pads.

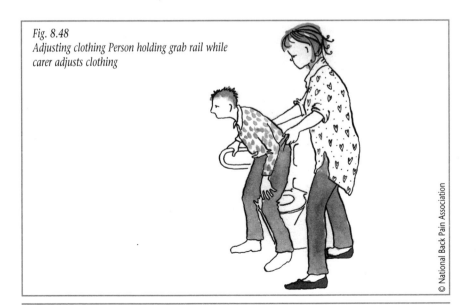

Fig. 8.48
Adjusting clothing Person holding grab rail while carer adjusts clothing

© National Back Pain Association

9.2.a. Person unable to weightbear

For a Person who is unable to weightbear, you need to consider bridging board transfers. The carer will also need to consider the use of a sling lifting hoist. You can use an 'access' or 'toileting' sling (see Chapter 6: Equipment) to provide easy access for adjusting clothing while the Person is still in the sling. However, this type of sling does not give good support so the Person will require good trunk control. If more support is required and a full sling is used, then the Person's clothing will need to be adjusted either after he has been transferred onto the toilet by rocking him side to side (similar to 8.3. above), or before the sling is put on (e.g. in bed). Cleaning may also need to take place back on the bed if a full sling is used. Be careful if a full sling is used, to protect the sling from soiling on the return journey to the bed.

A carer is not a grab rail nor a hoist and should not be used as one!

9.2.b. Special considerations when assisting people to use the toilet

♦ Warn the Person not to push or pull on unstable surfaces such as sinks, taps and toilet roll holders, or to use the carer as a grab rail or hoist.

♦ Consider the use of automatic cleaning and drying toilet systems.

♦ Cleaning a Person in a sitting or standing position requires prior assessment of him and his ability as well as the space available. Cleaning could be done as follows:

Fig. 8.49
Person leaning forward and carer cleaning (back in normal upright position)

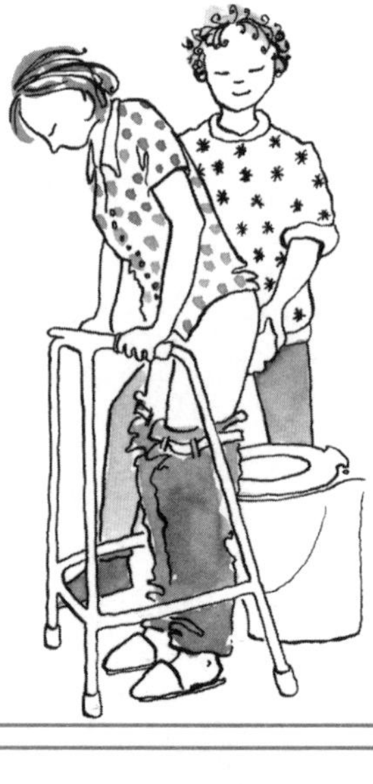

© National Back Pain Association

♦ Encourage the Person to clean himself. Gloves may be helpful if the Person has difficulty with co-ordination.

♦ Ensure the Person can reach the toilet paper and can tear a piece from the roll. If not, ready folded sheets may be more useful or a device which automatically tears the paper.

♦ Asking the Person to lean from one side to the other or to lean forwards will provide access for the carer. An additional carer may be required to assist with supporting the Person when he is leaning forward.

♦ Hoist the Person back onto bed onto a towel or disposable pad then clean and redress him.

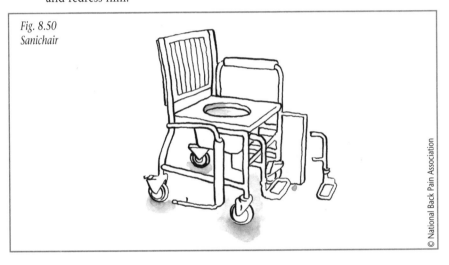

Fig. 8.50
Sanichair

© National Back Pain Association

♦ If access to the toilet is restricted, then transfer the Person onto a wheeled commode (Fig. 8.50) and either push this over a standard toilet or use it in an area where there is more space.

♦ It may be helpful to modify these transfers and positions for people who have upper limb strength but problems with the use of lower limbs (e.g. bilateral leg amputee or paralysis). This Person could transfer onto the toilet forwards facing the cistern with their lower limbs or stumps astride the toilet pan (Fig. 8.51).

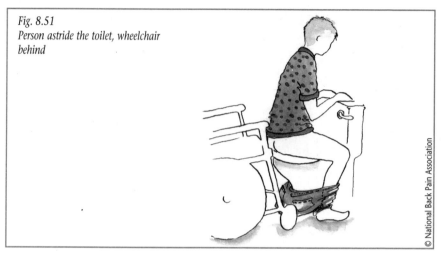

Fig. 8.51
Person astride the toilet, wheelchair behind

© National Back Pain Association

♦ If a Person is using a bridging board he may find it more difficult once clothing is removed. If talcum powder is sprinkled onto the board, friction will be reduced but the risk of the movement becoming less controlled and the Person slipping off the board is increased and this is, therefore, not recommended. An incontinence pad, with plastic side up, may also help reduce the friction between the Person's skin and the board, but the safest method is to adjust clothing once on the toilet.

♦ It is important to follow safety and hygiene procedures when assisting People to use the toilet. Gloves and aprons should be provided and care taken when emptying commodes. Regular emptying of the pan will prevent lifting of a heavy, unstable load. To avoid spilling the contents when emptying a chemical commode, carers should avoid carrying full pans over long distances or up and down stairs. More visits to a Person may be required if the commode fills up quickly. The carer must take care to observe basic handling principles when lifting and replacing chemical commodes. Deal with any spillages safely and hygienically.

Never use the Underarm Drag Lift, Pivot Transfer, Bear Hug or any other transfer involving a carer taking the full or most of the weight of the Person being transferred onto or off the toilet (see Section 11 below).

9.3 UNSAFE TECHNIQUES (See also Section 11)

- ⊗ UNSAFE TECHNIQUE - UNDERARM DRAG LIFT OR ANY VERSION OF IT
- ⊗ UNSAFE TECHNIQUE - PIVOT TRANSFER / BEAR HUG / STANDING TRANSFER
- ⊗ UNSAFE TECHNIQUE - TAKING ALL OR MOST OF THE WEIGHT OF THE PERSON BEING TRANSFERRED
- ⊗ UNSAFE TECHNIQUE - USING THE CARER AS A GRAB RAIL OR HOIST
- ⊗ UNSAFE TECHNIQUE - TRYING TO HOLD A PERSON UPRIGHT WHILE PROVIDING PERSONAL OR HYGIENE CARE

10. Special situations

Special situations in the community are too many and varied to give individual guidance and, like the other portions of this chapter and book, the advice is broadly based and each situation must be judged on its own merits following a full assessment. The following guidance is not to be taken on its own but used in conjunction with other information provided in this book and appropriate manual handling training prior to using the techniques.

In all special situations the following approach is recommended.

- ♦ **ASSESS** Don't just rush headlong into the situation; look at all the circumstances surrounding. Based on the assessment you should:

- ♦ **PLAN** What you intend to do and the things that must be done first to lower the risks to the lowest level reasonably practicable. Then follow the guide of:

- ♦ **MINIMAL HANDLING** - You physically move the Person only if no other method is appropriate based on your assessment.

10.1. ELDERLY PEOPLE

There are certain problems and diseases associated with the ageing process but just because someone is elderly does not mean they will resist the use of equipment more than others; or that they are more anxious or agitated than other people in similar circumstances; or that they may suddenly fail to stand any more than anyone else when they have consistently stood previously. Care needs should be assessed on an individual basis. In other words, being elderly does not present any extra special care problems more so than may be encountered in the general population.

10.2. REFUSAL TO USE APPROPRIATE EQUIPMENT

If a Person refuses to be moved with equipment which is necessary for safety, he must not be moved. You need to investigate why he has refused. Time invested explaining equipment, its features, benefits and reasons for use, before introducing the equipment itself, will frequently reassure the Person (see Chapter 5: The Person and the environment).

Other areas to investigate include: Is the carer herself reluctant to use it? Her anxiety about the use of equipment will be picked up by the Person. Are the items of equipment and any attachments clean? Stained or soiled slings on a hoist will affect a Person's willingness to use it. Has the Person had an unpleasant previous experience with the equipment or the carer's ability to use it? If a carer has been poorly trained, or not trained at all on equipment, she may fit it and/or use it inappropriately causing the Person discomfort. If all avenues have been explored and explained and the Person still refuses to use the equipment then he should not be moved from the bed. All nursing and personal care should be provided in bed until the Person is prepared to use the appropriate equipment (see Chapter 5: The Person and the environment).

10.3. UNCONSCIOUS PERSON

The unconscious Person may be someone in long-term care provided in the home or in a nursing home. A high level of care is needed; an in-depth assessment will determine the number of carers required and appropriate equipment to reduce the level of risk involved with manually handling the unconscious Person. Supine (lying down) transfers should be used for moves up and down the bed, as well as laterally on and off shower trolleys etc. A profiling bed and a hoist should be basic equipment for these moves as well as padded turning sheets to turn the Person onto his side. At all times respect for the dignity of the Person should be maintained. It is important to speak to an unconscious Person and inform him of what is about to occur or is occurring; although an unconscious Person cannot give feedback, he needs the same information as a conscious Person.

10.4. PERSON FAILING TO STAND UNEXPECTEDLY

At times a Person who has been capable of standing with or without assistance may suddenly fail to stand when the carer expects him to. The carer should not allow any further attempts to stand until a full reassessment has been carried out to find the reason. Was this a one-off occurrence or has the Person's physical or mental state deteriorated? If it is not a one-off episode, see Section 1 above for guidance. All other carers who may be involved in assisting the Person to stand need to know and should be informed. Make a record of the occurrence, reassessment findings and new moving and handling recommendations in the Person's care plan (PHP) (See Chapter 3: Assessing risks).

10.5. PERSON WITH SPECIAL NEEDS (INCLUDING LEARNING AND/OR PHYSICAL DIFFICULTIES)

It is essential to enable a Person with special needs to have a meaningful quality of life. Their right to this is the same as anyone else in society. Many of the moving and handling techniques noted in this chapter are appropriate for People with special needs but a detailed discussion is beyond the scope of this book. The reader is referred to the Further Reading section at the end of the chapter for further information and guidance.

10.6. PERSON WITH INVOLUNTARY MOVEMENTS (E.G. MUSCLE SPASMS)

Many involuntary movements are aggravated by inappropriate moving and handling techniques or holds. They may also be exacerbated if the Person: is cold or anxious, has to deal with something new (e.g. a new carer or changed environment) or when the Person is held. In all instances, specialist advice should be sought from a therapist with experience of moving People who have some neurological impairment. Specialist advice may include, for example, a pre-medication (e.g. a Person with Parkinson's Disease may have their medication regime altered to allow the medication time to take effect before morning personal care is provided), or having the Person initiate the movement and the carer co-ordinating her movement with the Person's movements.

10.7. PERSON COLLAPSED IN RESTRICTED SPACE/AREA

STOP! If you have come across a Person on the floor or ground and did not witness the event that brought them to the ground, then firstly follow the guidance for approaching a fallen Person (see above Section 7.1).

After this has been done and once sufficient help has arrived, the carer can then follow the steps below.

- Turn the Person onto his side (see 3.1. above).

- Insert a low friction roller or sliding device fitted with extension straps.

- Turn the Person in the other direction and finish inserting the sliding device with extension straps.

- The carers stand and position in a walk stance by the side by the Person and firmly grasp the extension straps.

- One carer says clearly 'Ready, Steady, Slide' and, on the word 'Slide', both carers walk backwards pulling the extension straps with them allowing the Person to be slid out into a clear area where a hoist should then be used to bring him up from the floor.

10.8. PERSON COLLAPSED OUTDOORS

STOP! If you have come across a Person on the floor or ground and did not witness the event that brought them to the ground, then firstly follow the guidance for approaching a fallen Person (see above Section 7.1). Make the area safe first.

- Dial 999.

- Carry out First Aid as needed.

10.9. A PERSON WITH DEMENTIA

- See 2.2.a. above.

10.10. PERSON WHO SITS DOWN BEFORE REACHING THE DESTINATION

- Stay close to the Person.

- Follow them with a chair. OR

- Use a handling belt with your feet in position ready to help the Person sit down.

- A second or third carer can be ready to push a chair underneath the Person if/when he sits down too soon.

10.11. TERMINALLY ILL PERSON

Following assessment, many of the techniques described above will be appropriate for a Person who is terminally ill and, when used correctly, they will maximise the comfort while caring for him. Confidence in using the appropriate techniques will help to lessen any pressure that may be put on the carer by the family to use unsafe and uncomfortable techniques. As with the unconscious Person, the terminally ill Person should be treated with respect and dignity at all times. Speak to them informing them of what is about to occur or is occurring and the reasons for it.

11. Unsafe techniques

11.1 'AUSTRALIAN' OR SHOULDER LIFT (OR SHOULDER SLIDE) (Fig. 8.52)

The use of this lift has been a leading cause of injuries in nurses (RCN, 1996). The Person being moved using this method was substantially to the side and behind the carer with his arms down her back. One of the carer's arms was held twisted and gripped by the other carer underneath the Person's thighs. The near arm and shoulder of the carer took the full weight of the Person and transferred it in an uneven fashion through the shoulders to the carer's other arm and hand braced on the bed acting as a pivot. In effect, the full weight of the Person was transferred unevenly from one arm and shoulder to the other acting as a pivot. The variation of the pivot hand holding the Person's back instead of being placed on the bed increased the risk still further. Another variation used sliding devices placed underneath the Person's bottom to 'slide' him up. The carer still had to transfer the full weight of the Person through the shoulders as described.

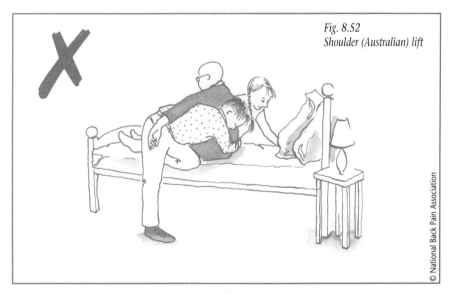

*Fig. 8.52
Shoulder (Australian) lift*

© National Back Pain Association

11.2 ORTHODOX OR CRADLE LIFT (Figs. 8.53 and 8.54)

This lift has been the second most common cause of injuries in nurses (RCN, 1996). Two carers stood either side of the bed, locked hands under the Person's shoulder and lower back/buttocks then lifted, twisting their backs while stooping forward holding the full weight of the Person and then set the Person down further up in the bed.

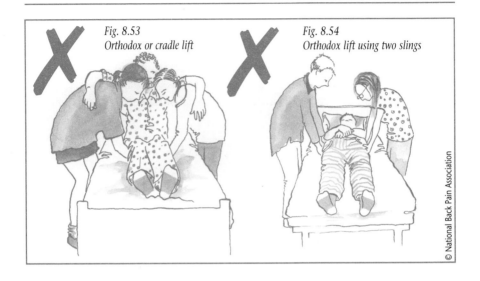

Fig. 8.53
Orthodox or cradle lift

Fig. 8.54
Orthodox lift using two slings

© National Back Pain Association

11.3 FLIP TURN (Fig. 8.55)

One or two carers stood on the same side of the bed and reached under the Person. Both simultaneously pulled the Person towards them while lifting and turning him onto his side. This technique was also inappropriately used to move a Person across the bed.

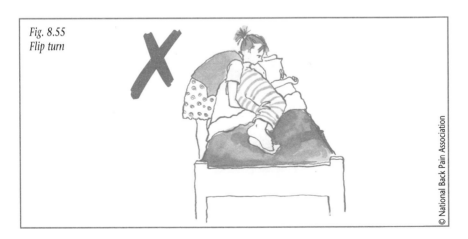

Fig. 8.55
Flip turn

© National Back Pain Association

11.4 UNDERARM DRAG LIFT (OR ANY VERSION OF IT) (Figs. 8.56, 8.57, 8.58 and 8.59)

This has been the fourth leading cause of injuries in nurses (RCN, 1996). Carers placed their hand or arm under the Person's axilla (armpit) and literally lifted by dragging the Person up. The lift was frequently used to drag people up from a chair/wheelchairs to stand, to transfer from one chair into another, move further up in bed etc.

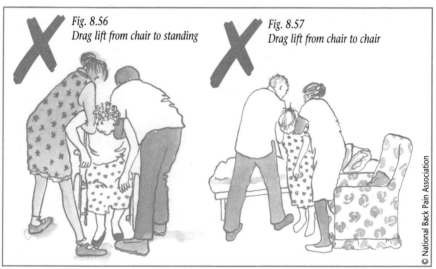

Fig. 8.56
Drag lift from chair to standing

Fig. 8.57
Drag lift from chair to chair

© National Back Pain Association

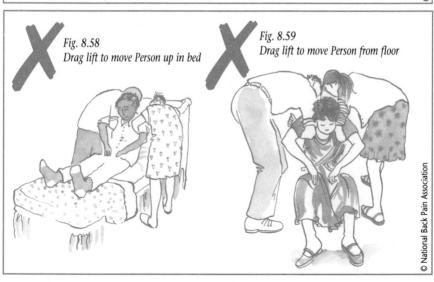

Fig. 8.58
Drag lift to move Person up in bed

Fig. 8.59
Drag lift to move Person from floor

© National Back Pain Association

11.5 STANDING IN FRONT OF A PERSON - PIVOT TRANSFER, ELBOW LIFT, BEAR HUG OR STANDING TRANSFER (Figs. 8.60, 8.61 and 8.62)

The Person held the carer either around the waist or the neck and, if the Person lost balance or collapsed, he would drag the carer down. The carer's posture was unsafe and she was not able to maintain the natural curves of the spine. These techniques required a lot of strength on the part of the carer and, once moving, the carer would find the manoeuvre difficult to control causing her to virtually 'throw' the Person into the chair to which they were going.

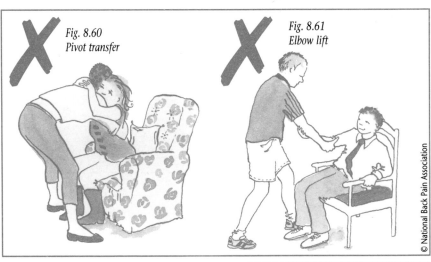

Fig. 8.60
Pivot transfer

Fig. 8.61
Elbow lift

© National Back Pain Association

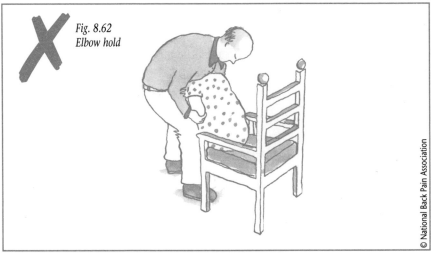

Fig. 8.62
Elbow hold

© National Back Pain Association

11.6 TOP AND TAIL (OR THROUGH-ARM LIFT) (Fig. 8.63)

Two carers were involved in this unsafe technique. One carer lifted from under the arms by locking her hands onto the Person's folded forearms and she took most of the Person's weight while bending forward. The carer lifting the feet was taking approximately 32% of the Person's body weight while stooping down and frequently twisting.

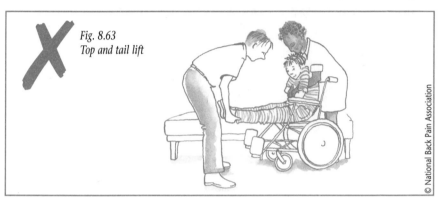

Fig. 8.63
Top and tail lift

© National Back Pain Association

11.7 POOR TEAM HANDLING

Team moving here refers to two, three, four or more carers physically moving a Person. When team lifting and carrying, the full weight of the Person was taken. An example of poor team handling is two, three or more carers trying to manually lift a Person up from the floor and carry them to a bed. The carers all had to use stooped postures holding the Person away from them when starting and finishing. Most beds in the community are low fixed-height beds which increase the stooping and reaching risks. Increasing numbers meant another hazard of increased difficulty, namely all carers starting and finishing the move at exactly the same time.

11.8 LIFTING INTO/OUT OF THE BATH

A Person standing barefoot on a wet slippery surface is unstable and in this situation the risks to both the Person and the carer are dramatically increased. If the carer was taking the full weight of a Person getting into or out of the bath and the Person slipped, this would result in the full weight of the Person suddenly being thrown onto the carer. Lifting into or out of the bath using through arm holds (Fig. 8.64) or underarm drags had the same high risk factors as outlined above (11.4 and 11.6) plus the added problems of wet slippery surfaces.

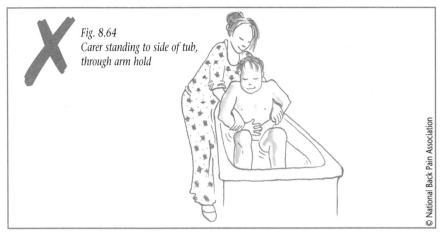

Fig. 8.64
Carer standing to side of tub, through arm hold

© National Back Pain Association

11.9 USING FLEXION (Figs. 8.65 a-c)

Knees straight and back bent put extra stress on the spine unnecessarily. An added twist while flexing increases the risks of injury to the carer. The instances where flexion is used are numerous but a few examples include repositioning a Person's feet (Fig. 8.65a), assisting with feeding (Fig. 8.65b) and talking to a Person (Fig. 8.65c).

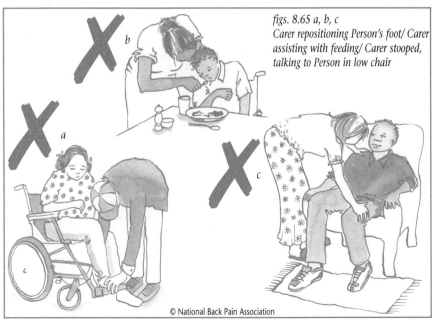

figs. 8.65 a, b, c
Carer repositioning Person's foot/ Carer assisting with feeding/ Carer stooped, talking to Person in low chair

© National Back Pain Association

11.10 TRYING TO HOLD A PERSON UPRIGHT WHILE PROVIDING PERSONAL OR HYGIENE CARE (Fig. 8.66)

If one carer tried to steady a Person standing upright while providing personal or hygiene care, this allowed the Person to hold the carer around either the waist or neck while the carer used one hand to steady the Person and the other hand to provide hygiene care, while simultaneously twisting and using flexion.

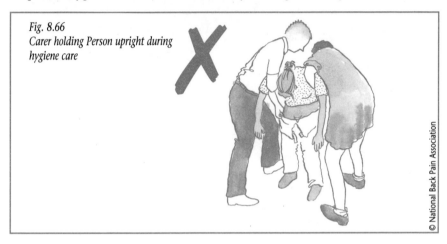

Fig. 8.66
Carer holding Person upright during hygiene care

© National Back Pain Association

11.11 ARM AND LEG LUG (Fig. 8.67)

Two carers each gripped the Person's upper arms and thighs thus taking the full weight while in flexion and using twisting motions.

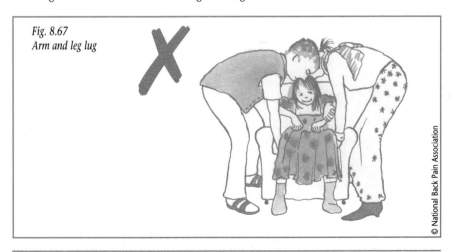

Fig. 8.67
Arm and leg lug

© National Back Pain Association

11.12 DRAG LIFT WITH HANDLING SLING

Similar to usual Drag Lift.

11.13 CROSS ARM LIFT

Two carers held the Person under the arms and were twisting while lifting the full weight of the Person using a handling sling placed under the Person's bottom.

11.14 TAKING ALL OR MOST OF THE WEIGHT OF THE PERSON

Excess weight.

11.15 USING THE CARER AS A GRAB RAIL OR HOIST

Unstable or collapsing Person would drag the carer or cause a sudden jerk on her spine.

11.16 PERSON WITH ARMS AROUND CARER'S NECK OR WAIST

Unstable or collapsing Person would drag the carer or cause sudden jerk on her spine.

11.17 THREE CARER LIFT AND CARRY TROLLEY TO BED

Same as Team handling (11.7) above.

11.18 CANVAS AND POLES

The carer was taking the full weight of a Person while holding the Person away from her and using flexion and twisting motions.

11.19 USING LINEN SHEETS TO LIFT OR DRAG

Sheets would rip and tear.

11.20 PUSHING THE PERSON'S FEET FORWARD BY THE CARER USING HER FOOT

Person not capable of walking.

11.21 WALKING PERSON WITH HISTORY OF FREQUENT FALLS

A falling Person identified as high risk many times.

11.22 USING TWO SLINGS TO LIFT

Both carers, therefore, were taking the full weight of the Person.

11.23 ROCKING TRANSFER WITH TWO CARERS

The carer stood in front of the Person and adopted poor postures and had to twist; the carer standing behind Person in poor posture had to reach and stretch while in flexion then twist.

REFERENCES

Campbell, R.J., (1996). Psychiatric Dictionary, Seventh Edition. Oxford University Press, Oxford/New York.

Disabled Living Foundation, (1994). Handling People: Equipment, advice and information. Disabled Living Foundation, London.

National Back Pain Association, (1998). The Guide to the Handling of Patients, Fourth Edition. National Back Pain Association in collaboration with the Royal College of Nursing, London.

RCN, (1996). Hazards of Nursing, Personal Injuries at Work. RCN, London.

Unreported, (1987). Bayley v. Bloomsbury Health Authority. Mr Justice Henry, Royal Courts of Justice, 1985. B No. 531.

FURTHER INFORMATION ON SPECIAL NEEDS

Brown, R.I., (1997). Quality of Life for People With Disabilities, Second Edition. Stanley Thornes, Cheltenham. (Available from DfEE.)

Gastrell, P. and Edwards, J. (Eds), (1997). Community Health Nursing, Frameworks for Practice, Bailliere Tindall, London.

Kenrick, M. and Luker, K.A., (Eds), (1995). Clinical Nursing Practice in the Community, Blackwell Science Berlin, Germany.

Tully, K., (1986). Improving Residential Life for Disabled. Churchill Livingstone, London.

9 Further Information

Age Concern England
Astral House
1268 London Road
London SW16 4ER
Telephone: 020 8679 8000
Website: www.ace.org.uk

Alzheimers' Disease Society
Gordon House
10 Greencoat Place
London SW1P 1PH
Telephone: 020 7306 0606
e-mail: info@alzheimers.org.uk
Website: www.alzheimers.org.uk

Arthritis Care
18 Stephenson Way
London NW1 3HD
Telephone: 020 7916 1500
Website: www.arthritiscare.org.uk

BackCare
16 Elmtree Road
Teddington
Middlesex TW11 8ST
Telephone: 020 8977 5474
e-mail: backcare@compuserve.com
Website: www.backcare.org.uk

British Heart Foundation
14 Fitzhardinge Street
London W1H 4DH
Telephone: 020 7935 0185
Website: www.bhf.org.uk

Carers National Association
Ruth Pitter House
20-25 Glasshouse Yard
London EC1A 4JS
Telephone: 020 7490 8818
Carers line: 0345 573369
e-mail: internet@ukcarers.org
Website: www.carersuk.demon.co.uk

Chest, Heart and Stroke Association
63 North Castle Street
Edinburgh
EH2 3LT
Telephone: 0131 225 6963
e-mail: chss@del.pipex.com

Disabled Living Foundation
380-384 Harrow Road
London W9 2HU
Telephone: 020 7289 6111
Helpline: 0870 603 9177
Minicom: 0870 603 9176
e-mail: dlfinfo@dlf.org.uk
Website: www.dlf.org.uk

MENCAP - The Royal Society for Mentally Handicapped Children & Adults
123 Golden Lane
London EC1Y 0RT
Telephone: 020 7454 0454
Website: www.mencap.org.uk

MIND - The National Association for Mental Health

15-19 The Broadway
Stratford
London E15 4BQ
Telephone: 020 8519 2122
e-mail: contact@mind.org.uk
Website: www.mind.org.uk

Multiple Sclerosis Society of Great Britain and Northern Ireland

25 Effie Road
Fulham
London SW6 1EE
Telephone: 020 7610 7171
e-mail: info@mssociety.org.uk
Website: www.mssociety.org.uk

National Association of Citizens Advice Bureaux

Myddleton House
115-123 Pentonville Road
London N1 9LZ
Telephone: 020 7833 2181
e-mail: consultancy@nacab.org.uk
Website: www.nacab.org.uk

National Schizophrenia Fellowship

28 Castle Street
Kingston upon Thames
Surrey KT1 1SS
Telephone: 020 8 547 3937
e-mail: info@nsf.org.uk
Website: www.nsf.org.uk

Parkinson's Disease Society of the UK

22 Upper Woburn Place
London WC1H 0RA
Telephone: 020 7931 8080
e-mail: mailbox@pdsuk.demon.co.uk

Relatives Association
5 Tavistock Place
London WC1H 9SN
Telephone: 020 7692 4302

Royal Association for Disability and Rehabilitation (RADAR)
12 City Forum
250 City Road
London EC1V 8AF
Telephone: 020 7250 3222
e-mail: radar@radar.org.uk
Website: www.radar.org.uk

Royal National Institute for the Blind (RNIB)
224 Great Portland Street
London W1N 6AA
Telephone: 020 7388 1266
e-mail: (contact name)@rnib.org.uk
Website: www.rnib.org

Royal National Institute for the Deaf (RNID)
19-23 Featherstone Street
London EC1Y 8SL
Telephone: 020 7296 8000/8001
Website: www.rnid.org.uk

SANE - Schizophrenia - A National Emergency
1st Floor
Cityside House
40 Alder Street
London E1 1EE
Telephone: 020 7375 1002
Website: www.mkn.co.uk/help/charity/sane/index

Glossary

Atrophy
wasting away of body tissue (muscles or organs) caused through lack of use

Biomechanics
the study of forces on the human body

Cognitive
refers to the ability of human beings to know and understand things. Used in Chapter 8 to describe 'dementia' - a 'cognitive disorder'. This condition affects an individual's awareness and perception of the world around them.

Compression
the force resulting from two surfaces being pressed together

Ergonomics
getting the best 'fit' between people and the things they do and the equipment they use

Key worker
a person who acts as the main point of contact or reference within an organisation

Mother tongue
one's first or native language

Shear (shearing effect)
the force resulting when two surfaces in contact with each other are moved or slid across one another

Index

*Note: Page numbers in **bold** type indicate illustrations*